Recovering After A Stroke

A Comprehensive Guide To Stroke Recovery Through Neuroplasticity And Nutrition

Dr. Benjamin Sterling

© **Copyright 2024 - All rights reserved.**

The content contained within this book may not be reproduced, duplicated or transmitted without direct written permission from the author or the publisher.

Under no circumstances will any blame or legal responsibility be held against the publisher, or author, for any damages, reparation, or monetary loss due to the information contained within this book, either directly or indirectly.

Legal Notice:

This book is copyright protected. It is only for personal use. You cannot amend, distribute, sell, use, quote or paraphrase any part, or the content within this book, without the consent of the author or publisher.

Disclaimer Notice:

Please note the information contained within this document is for educational and entertainment purposes only. All effort has been executed to present accurate, up to date, reliable, complete information. No warranties of any kind are declared or implied. Readers acknowledge that the author is not engaged in the rendering of legal, financial, medical or professional advice. The content within this book has been derived from various sources. Please consult a licensed professional before attempting any techniques outlined in this book.

By reading this document, the reader agrees that under no circumstances is the author responsible for any losses, direct or indirect, that are incurred as a result of the use of the information contained within this document, including, but not limited to, errors, omissions, or inaccuracies.

Contents

Introduction 1

1. The Science Behind Neuroplasticity 7
   The Brain's Amazing Ability to Recover: A Look at Neuroplasticity
   Adaptability Across Lifespan
   Factors Influencing Neuroplasticity
   How Neuroplasticity Works in Stroke Recovery and Recovery
   Brain Boosting Foods

2. Building a Foundation for Optimized Recovery 19
   Understanding Your Stroke and Its Implications
   Stroke Types
   Evaluating the Stroke Symptoms
   Neuroplasticity and Stroke
   Assembling Your Healthcare Team - Roles and Expectations
   Identifying the Who and Why of Your Team
   Long and Short-Term Monitoring
   What Does Recovery Look Like?
   Emotional Resilience in the Face of Adversity

      Stress Management: Coping with the Recovery

3. Nutrition and Stroke   33
      The Connection Between Nutrition and Brain Health
      Long-term Benefits of Eating Healthy
      Nutrients to Aid Stroke Recovery
      Staying Hydrated
      Role of Nutrition in Stroke Recovery
      Impact of Sodium
      Examples of Diet Plans

4. Integrating Neuroplasticity and Diet   51
      Exploring the Synergy Between Neuroplasticity and Our Diet
      Mindful Eating
      Neuroplastic Eating Recommendations

5. Physical Rehabilitation Strategies   63
      Goal Setting Post Stroke
      Physiotherapy Techniques for Strengthening and Mobility
      Physiotherapy Exercise Regimens
      Occupational Therapy Strategies for Daily Life Skills
      Environmental Adjustments or Modifications
      Use of Speech and Language Therapy
      Non-Traditional Therapies to Consider

6. Cognitive Rehabilitation Strategies   79
      Rebuilding Memory Function Post-Stroke
      Memory Exercises
      Memory Strategies
      Improving Attention and Concentration
      How to Improve Concentration
      Creating a Safe Environment

7. Psychological Well-being After a Stroke — 95
   Dealing with Anxiety and Depression Post-Stroke
   Depression
   Anxiety
   Understanding Personality Changes
   Managing Stress

8. Lifestyle Modifications for Optimal Health — 107
   Adopting a Heart-Healthy Diet
   Exercise Plan
   Sleep

9. Prevention Of Future Strokes — 121
   Identifying and Managing Risks
   Lifestyle Modifications
   Celebrating Milestones and Gains
   Tracking Progress and Goals
   Medications
   Physicals
   Continuing Your Recovery

10. Living a Fulfilling Life Post-Stroke — 131
    Reclaiming Independence
    How Others Can Support

11. The Future of Stroke Recovery — 143
    Evolution of Technology in Stroke Recovery
    Understanding Genetics

Conclusion — 159

References — 163

Introduction

Start thinking wellness, not illness.
—Kate Allatt, Stroke Survivor

As a vibrant and cheerful man in his early fifties, I am passionate about hiking, painting, and parenting. One warm but windy Saturday morning, while on a morning hike with my family, I suddenly fell on my knees and collapsed. The right side of my body was numb, and I was unable to move it or speak coherently and audibly. Airlifted off the hiking trail by an emergency services helicopter, I arrived at Tampa General Hospital in Florida, where I was instantly diagnosed with a severe ischemic stroke.

My path to recovery was difficult, but I confronted all the challenges with conviction and a positive attitude. With the help of my family and a reliable team of healthcare experts, my rehabilitation began. At first, I grappled with easy tasks, such as grasping objects or building coherent word structures and sentences. However, I was resilient, propelling myself towards recovery through the drawbacks and frustration.

Over the following months, my progress was outstanding. By engaging in intensive occupational, physical, and speech therapy, I rediscovered the strength and mobility required to make my right side functional again and slowly improved my cognitive and speech abilities. My desire to recover, fueled by the support I received from my loved ones, drove my determination to regain the autonomy I had lost and get back to doing the activities I loved.

A year later, after that near-fatal stroke, I stood at the apex of my favorite hiking trail, tears of joy trickling down my cheeks. Despite having traveled a difficult path, I came out stronger, with more resilience than ever before. Up to this day, I still paint, hike, and spend quality time with my children. I try to instill within them a mindset of perseverance while inspiring people who face the same predicament to achieve their recovery goals.

Everything I have gone through is reminiscent of Kate Allatt, quoted at the beginning of this section. Kate Allatt's words encapsulate a life-changing shift in perspective that encourages individuals to prioritize proactive measures for overall health and well-being. Rather than fixate on the restrictions imposed by injury and illness, it promotes a focus on embracing a lifestyle that encourages mental, physical, and emotional health. For stroke survivors and others confronting health issues, this shift in thinking involves accepting rehabilitation, healthy habits, and self-care that promotes recovery and improves quality of life. By embracing a wellness-oriented frame of mind, you can regain a sense of urgency over your health, particularly the condition of your heart. You will become more resilient and empowered with a renewed acknowledgment of the chance to live a fulfilling life that transcends sickness (Allatt, 2013).

A stroke is a condition experienced when blood flow to a specific part of the brain is restricted or interrupted, resulting in damage suffered by the brain cells. This can lead to several neurological symptoms, like paralysis, speech impediments, or limited vision, depending on which part of the brain has been impacted. Strokes can be triggered by a blood clot that blocks a blood vessel (ischemic stroke) or by the rupture of a blood vessel (hemorrhagic stroke). Detecting the problem earlier is always ideal because you will receive the correct treatment plan to reduce long-term complications and improve results.

As a survivor of a stroke or an individual who is interested in obtaining knowledge on how one can recover from such a predicament, you are likely trying to learn several key aspects, such as:

1. **Rehabilitation techniques:** You probably want to learn about successful rehabilitation methods and therapies to reclaim emotional, physical, and cognitive function after experiencing a stroke.

2. **Managing symptoms:** You might seek guidance on controlling common post-stroke symptoms, such as weakness, speech challenges, cognitive impairments, and emotional changes.

3. **Preventing recurrence:** Mastering strategies to avoid future strokes and mitigate risk factors like diabetes, high blood pressure, and high cholesterol is vital for long-term recovery and good health.

4. **Support systems**: As a stroke survivor or caregiver, you might be interested in understanding the support systems available, such as home care, support groups, and resources for navigating the healthcare system.

In general, you are reading this book because you seek comprehensive guidance and practical advice on the complex and intricate path of stroke recovery, reclaiming your autonomy, and surviving a fulfilling life post-stroke.

Even some celebrities have suffered from strokes. Let's now turn our attention to some good examples of notable individuals who have openly revealed their experiences of surviving and bouncing back from a stroke:

- **Sharon Stone:** The vivacious and glamorous actress, who produced box office hits such as Basic Instinct, suffered a major stroke in 2001 at the relatively young age of 43. Initially, having been incapable of walking or talking, she had to go through intensive rehabilitation that finally enabled her to make a triumphant recovery. As soon as she had completed her rehab program, she instantly went back to her acting career and became an advocate for stroke awareness and prevention.

- **Kirk Douglas:** The actor, well-known for his roles in films like Spartacus and Paths of Glory, suffered a stroke in 1996 at the age of 80. However, Kirk was tough enough to battle the condition through rehabilitation and went on to lead a happy life, even making public appearances in his final years.

- **Dick Clark:** Another senior citizen who suffered a stroke in his late years is the legendary television host and producer Dick Clark. In 2004, at the age of 75, he underwent comprehensive rehabilitation and successfully bounced back to hosting duties, showcasing resilience and willpower in his recovery path.

The narratives of these famous people serve as motivational tales of survival and hope for you and a lot of other victims of strokes globally, suggesting that early detection, perseverance, and rehabilitation under conditions of adversity are essential traits to have when fighting against a stroke.

As the author, I am a physician specializing in stroke recovery and rehabilitation. I have over 20 years of experience in helping patients navigate the complex road to recovery after a stroke. My approach is deeply compassionate, leveraging the latest research to empower my patients to take charge of their recovery. I am passionate about sharing my knowledge and experiences to help stroke survivors regain control of their lives post-recovery. The experience and educational background I have in stroke management make me a highly competent individual to help you understand how to survive and recover from a stroke. Now that you have a brief understanding of a stroke, it is imperative to go into more detail on the subject; start by learning the science behind neuroplasticity in Chapter 1.

THE SCIENCE BEHIND NEUROPLASTICITY

This initial chapter takes you through the intricate workings of neuroplasticity, the brain's fantastic ability to rewire and adjust itself in response to a particular situation. It also helps you understand its significance in recovering from a stroke, illustrating the revolutionary processes essential to rehabilitation.

At one time, the medical field assumed that neuroplasticity was limited to early development; however, it is now seen as a long-term phenomenon. Neuroplasticity is the brain's ability to rewire itself in reaction to learning, experiences, and injury. By creating brand-new neural links and altering existing ones, the brain adapts to its environment (Puderbaugh & Emmady, 2023).

Based on information gained from cutting-edge studies, I will unravel the mechanisms fueling neuroplasticity. From synaptic plasticity (conditions in which relationships between neurons are weakened or strengthened) to neurogenesis (the formation of new neurons), every process leads to the brain's malleability. I will also unveil the critical role of gene expression, neurotransmitters, and growth factors in enabling these complicated alterations.

The Brain's Amazing Ability to Recover: A Look at Neuroplasticity

Neuroplasticity defines your ability to acquire new techniques, heal after suffering trauma to the brain, and embrace changes occurring in your environment. It is a process managed by intricate molecular and cellular systems, such as synaptic plasticity, neurogenesis, and alterations in neural connectivity. A good appreciation for neuroplasticity enlightens you on the brain's adaptive and resilient capacity, paving the way for creative interventions and therapies in rehabilitation and neuroscience (Puderbaugh & Emmady, 2023).

Adaptability Across Lifespan

Neuroplasticity is the ability to adapt across your lifespan, indicating the brain's outstanding capacity to restructure its function and components as a reaction to shifting demands and experiences. In early development stages, neuroplasticity enables fast learning and easy skills acquisition while your brain creates vital connections and refines neural circuits. This formative plasticity makes you develop the ability to acquire language, motor skills, and social behaviors, laying the platform for future cognitive abilities.

During adulthood, you will experience neuroplasticity, but in a more nuanced manner. While the brain's ability to foster rapid rewiring might diminish, it maintains its adaptability, continually restructuring in reaction to learning, environmental stimuli, and even injury. This long-term adaptability allows you to obtain new skills, reconfigure current ones, and successfully navigate complicated situations.

However, getting old can bring new challenges to neuroplasticity. Certain brain composition and function aspects might decline as you age, potentially affecting cognitive capacities and motor function. Nonetheless, research indicates that engaging in mentally stimulating actions, adhering to a healthy lifestyle, and engaging in lifelong learning can encourage neuroplasticity and mitigate the risks associated with age-related changes (Puderbaugh & Emmady, 2023).

Factors Influencing Neuroplasticity

Many factors impact neuroplasticity, fine-tuning the brain's capacity to adapt and restructure throughout life.

- **Environmental enrichment:** Exposure to a vibrant environment endowed with cognitive, sensory, and social experiences furthers neuroplasticity. Social relationships, novel stimuli, and learning opportunities create new neural bonds and enhance synaptic power.

- **Learning and experience:** Participating in complex and mentally challenging activities, such as learning a new technique or language, enables neuroplasticity. Learning induces synaptic connectivity changes and promotes the growth of new neurons, facilitating adaptive responses to new information and experiences.

- **Physical activity:** Constant workouts create ideal conditions for neuroplasticity because they enhance blood flow to the brain, encourage the release of neurotrophic factors, and help develop new neurons. Exercises, like aerobic workouts, are known for improving cognitive function and enabling brain health (Puderbaugh & Emmady, 2023).

- **Nutrition:** A balanced menu abundant in vital nutrients, antioxidants, and omega-3 fatty acids is good for brain health and neuroplasticity. Specific dietary elements, such as flavonoids obtained in fruits and vegetables, have increased synaptic plasticity and cognitive function.

- **Stress and emotional state:** Chronic stress might disrupt neuroplasticity by impairing synaptic connectivity and disturbing neurogenesis. On the other hand, positive emotions and social support may improve neuroplasticity and further resilience under adverse conditions.

By acknowledging these aspects, you can embrace lifestyle practices and interventions that help and improve neuroplasticity, encouraging brain health and cognitive function across your lifespan.

How Neuroplasticity Works in Stroke Recovery and Recovery

After you suffer a stroke, your brain goes through a remarkable process of restructuring, which, as you have learned before, is known as neuroplasticity. This phenomenon occurs to facilitate recovery and mitigate the impact of the damage triggered by the stroke. This process includes several vital mechanisms:

- **Functional reorganization:** When a stroke injures brain tissue, nearby neurons usually adopt new roles to mitigate the lost ability. This action is known as functional reorganization and allows undamaged parts of the brain to inherit the responsibilities of the damaged components, making you regain lost capacities over time.

- **Synaptic plasticity:** In the aftermath of a stroke, the association between neurons, commonly known as synapses, goes through modifications in power and connectivity. Synaptic plasticity strengthens the brain's ability to adapt to new requirements and learning curves, furthering the formation of alternative neural pathways to bypass damaged parts of the brain.

- **Neurogenesis:** Regardless of the long-held assumptions that neurogenesis (the formation of new neurons) only takes place during formative years, new evidence points to the fact that specific regions of the adult brain, especially the hippocampus, sustain the ability to generate new neurons. Neurogenesis may contribute to recovery after a stroke by replenishing damaged neuronal populations and integrating them into existing neural circuits.

- **Axonal sprouting:** New branches grow from current neurons to form connections with neighboring neurons. This procedure creates alternative neural pathways that bypass areas affected by the stroke and reestablish functionality.

- **Functional Rehabilitation:** Participating in rehabilitation therapies that include physical, speech, and occupational therapy is important in encouraging neuroplasticity and enabling recovery after a stroke. These therapies provide structured exercises and activities designed to promote the reorganization of neural networks and enhance functional outcomes (Puderbaugh & Emmady, 2023).

Neuroplasticity enables the brain to adapt and rewire itself in response to a stroke, providing hope for recovery and restoring function in affected individuals. Through targeted interventions and rehabilitation strategies, individuals can capitalize on the brain's remarkable capacity for adaptation and maximize their recovery potential.

Rehabilitation Techniques

When recovering from a stroke, rehabilitation techniques capitalize on neuroplasticity, the brain's ability to reorganize and form new connections, to promote recovery. Here's how neuroplasticity works in stroke recovery and the rehabilitation techniques that harness its potential:

- **Constraint-Induced Movement Therapy (CIMT):** CIMT incorporates prolonged exercise with the plagued limb while restricting the use of the unharmed. By requiring more use of the injured limb, this method forces the brain to reconfigure itself and encourages the resumption of movement via neuroplastic modifications.

- **Task-Specific Training:** Rehabilitation programs stress the execution of activities needed for everyday living, including walking and object-grasping. Through neural plasticity, the mind responds to repeatedly being subjected to such tasks, sharpening physical abilities while improving operational capabilities.

- **Mirror Therapy:** Mirror therapy replicates mobility in the undamaged limb on the harmed limb, providing an impression of activity in the impacted limb. Using visual stimulation, mirror therapy stimulates the brain's muscular systems, activating neural networks and promoting the recovery of motor skills (Yoshimura, 2021).

- **Electrical Stimulation:** Specific areas of the brain associated with movement are activated with currents of electricity utilizing transcranial magnetic stimulation (TMS) and prefrontal direct current stimulation (TDCS). These techniques enhance motor skill recovery by altering the brain's activity while encouraging neuroplasticity.

- **Virtual Reality (VR) Therapy:** VR-based therapy programs enable stroke victims to immerse themselves in engaging activities. VR therapy increases neuroplastic modifications in the brain and enhances motor skill development by resembling events from the real world.

- **Constraint-Induced Aphasia Therapy:** This type of therapy restricts the application of symbolic means of interaction, such as handwriting or movements, to encourage oral language and communication restoration in stroke patients suffering from aphasia.

People who have had a stroke may use neuroscience to promote recovery and reinstate compromised functionality by combining different treatment methods with concentrated and ongoing training. By emphasizing specific neurological routes, these methods may maximize neurological outcomes throughout rehabilitation following a stroke and help rebuild the cerebral cortex.

Mindful Practices

Through intentional mindfulness focus, neuroplasticity can be practiced in everyday situations to promote resistance and mental wellness. Mindfulness behaviors facilitate plasticity by:

- **Mindful meditation:** Activities that focus on awareness allow individuals to be more aware of their current moment while developing the ability to embrace their thoughts, feelings, and sensations without casting criticism. Continued practice has been shown to change the makeup and functioning of the nervous system in ways that enhance focus, control emotions, and lessen stress (Puderbaugh & Emmady, 2023).

- **Concentrated focus:** By concentrating attentiveness on particular feelings, including the sensation of breathing or bodily sensations, mindfulness exercises help grow the brain pathways associated with focused thought and memory. This concentrated attention might enhance mental agility and thinking skills, promoting adaptive answers to obstacles in everyday activities.

- **Stress reduction:** Chronic stress may harm neuroplasticity by breaking connections between neurons and reducing neurogenesis. By inducing serenity while decreasing anxiety, mindful behaviors offer the ideal setting for neuroplastic modifications.

- **Emotional regulation:** By encouraging understanding of one's subjective feelings and helping create appropriate ways to cope, mindfulness-based treatments assist individuals in becoming more mentally and physically resilient. This elevated control of feelings is associated with neuroplasticity through adaptive alterations in brain cell performance and structure.

- **Sensory awareness:** Meditation activities heighten consciousness toward your senses of touch, sight, taste, hearing, and smell. Through the action of increased sensory arousal and increased sensory awareness, you can improve your understanding of the present while encouraging neural development (Puderbaugh & Emmady, 2023).

Applying mindful techniques to daily life provides opportunities to develop neuroplasticity and enable general brain health. By being more aware, you can tap into your brain's adaptive capacity, encourage cognitive resilience, and improve overall health.

Physical Exercise and Activities

Utilizing neuroplasticity in your daily life by undertaking workouts and activities is a successful way to enrich your brain and build resilience after a stroke. You can consider some of the following ways to engage in regular workouts to support neuroplasticity:

- **Promotes neurogenesis:** Physical exercise promotes the manufacture of brain-derived neurotrophic factor (BDNF), a protein that is helpful in the growth and survival of neurons. Elevated quantities of BDNF enhance neurogenesis, the birth of new neurons, especially in areas of the brain related to learning and memory, like the hippocampus.

- **Enhances synaptic plasticity:** As mentioned previously, exercise improves blood circulation to the mind, supplying oxygen and vital minerals required for neuronal operation. This increased blood movement helps synaptic plasticity, the capacity of neurons to create and strengthen links, thereby enabling learning and memory processes to work correctly (Puderbaugh & Emmady, 2023).

- **Improves cognitive function:** Frequent workouts have been known to enhance cognitive operation across many domains, such as memory, attention, and executive function. By enhancing neuroplastic alterations in the brain, workouts can improve neural effectiveness and maximize cognitive performance.

- **Reduces neuroinflammation:** Working out has an anti-inflammatory impact on your mind, lowering levels of pro-inflammatory cytokines and oxidative anxiety. By mitigating neuroinflammation, workouts build an environment suitable for neuroplasticity and support general brain wellness.

Regular physical exercise and activities in daily life provide numerous benefits for brain health and neuroplasticity. By staying active, individuals can optimize cognitive function, promote neuroplasticity, and support overall well-being.

Brain Boosting Foods

Consuming meals that contain essential vitamins and minerals that encourage brain wellness and memory retention is a single method of integrating neuroplasticity throughout everyday life via a mind-boosting diet. There are plenty of ways in which a healthy, nutrient-rich meal promotes neuroplasticity, and let's now explore some of the pertinent ones:

- **Omega-3 fatty acids:** The central nervous system fundamentally depends on omega-3 fats, especially EPA and DHA, present in oily fish like salmon, trout, and anchovies. These fatty acids enhance neuroplastic alterations in the cerebral cortex by encouraging the formation of new tissue, promoting synaptic flexibility, and enhancing neurotransmission.

- **Antioxidants:** Antioxidants, including vitamins C and E and flavonoids found in fruits, vegetables, and nuts, keep the human brain safe from inflammation and oxidative stress. They also offer an atmosphere beneficial for neuroplasticity and memory retention by eliminating harmful radicals and decreasing neurological inflammation.

- **B vitamins:** The manufacture of synapses and the function of the cerebral cortex depend on B vitamins, for example, B6, B12, and folate. B vitamin-rich nutrients can be found in green leafy vegetables, beans, eggs, and lean meats. These substances strengthen mental abilities and could boost neurogenesis by promoting the production of neurotransmitters essential for learning and recall (Puderbaugh & Emmady, 2023).

- **Polyphenols:** Berries, dark chocolate, and green leafy tea are some foodstuffs high in polyphenols, which possess neuroprotective and neuroplastic characteristics. These chemicals have been proven to enhance brain health, synaptic plasticity, memory, and cognition by altering neuronal development and survival signals.

- **Good fats:** Consuming healthy fats from products like almonds, avocados, and olive oil provides the cognitive system with the nutrition required to maintain its form and function. These kinds of lipids promote cellular stability.

Brain-boosting foods in daily meals and snacks can support neuroplasticity, enhance cognitive function, and promote overall brain health. Individuals can optimize their cognitive abilities and support lifelong learning and adaptation by nourishing the brain with essential nutrients.

The importance of factors related to lifestyle when assessing the durability and well-being of the cerebral cortex is demonstrated by neuroplasticity. Acquiring novel talents, keeping a physically active routine, and engaging in mindfulness are brain-stimulating endeavors that may increase neuroplasticity while improving overall health. With an extensive approach consisting of empirical studies, personalized treatments, and daily actions, scientists can fully realize the endless possibilities of neuroplasticity and allow folks to enjoy fulfilling lives that are improved by continuous growth, modification, and training. The foundation-building phase of optimum recovery will be addressed in the upcoming chapter.

Building a Foundation for Optimized Recovery

Your body is resistant to almost anything. It's your mind that you have to convince.

–Unknown

Healing after a stroke is an intricate procedure that includes both physical and mental components. Each development and achievement is a testament to the body's and mind's resilience. As the unidentified quotation implies, the brain is essential to this procedure.

This chapter examines the fundamental concepts of stroke recovery, emphasizing the importance of establishing a solid foundation for growth. We will explore how individuals can take an active role in their recovery process, from understanding the intricate nature of neuroplasticity to adopting an integrated approach.

Employing the latest discoveries in addition to viewpoints from survivors of strokes, caretakers, and medical professionals, we offer techniques and strategies meant to promote a setting that is perfect for complete recuperation. Each element—mental stimulation, rehabilitation, or emotional support—contributes significantly to fostering the brain-body link, essential for regaining independence and an excellent standard of living following a stroke.

While this study could prove challenging, it provides endless potential for growth and recovery. With determination, support, and a commitment to good health, you build the basis for a road to a full recovery, renewed confidence, and an increasingly hopeful post-stroke destiny.

Understanding Your Stroke and Its Implications

Learning what happened and how it impacts you following a stroke is crucial for finding out how you can feel better. The types and degrees of strokes can vary, each posing distinct challenges and factors to consider. By learning about the various kinds of strokes, individuals can make informed choices regarding their medical care and recovery and gain a greater understanding of their illness.

Stroke Types

- **Ischemic stroke:** This kind of stroke occurs when a clot of blood clogs or reduces the circumference of an artery responsible for delivering blood to the cerebral cortex. The majority of cases of strokes are ischemic, which might lead to several neurological injuries dependent on the size and location of the obstruction (WebMD, 2022),

- **Hemorrhagic stroke:** The following form of stroke is a hemorrhagic stroke that takes place when a blood vessel ruptures in any part of the brain, resulting in hemorrhage and subsequent injury to the adjacent brain tissue. Arteriovenous malformations (AVMs), aneurysms, as well as hypotension, are some of the few conditions that can lead to this kind of stroke. Since hemorrhagic strokes may result in possibly fatal repercussions, medical attention must occur immediately (WebMD, 2022).

- **Transient Ischemic Attack (TIA):** Often known as a "mini-stroke," a TIA occurs during a brief reduction in blood movement to the brain's cerebral cortex. While TIAs typically pass completely in a couple of minutes to hours, if disregarded, they enhance the likelihood of recurrent strokes and serve as warning signs of deeper cardiovascular issues (WebMD, 2022).

Knowing the distinctions between these types of strokes may assist patients in working closely with healthcare professionals to create customized therapies and preventive measures. Furthermore, being conscious of a stroke's impact on the brain, body, or feelings allows anyone to take steps to satisfy their own needs and optimize their recovery process.

Evaluating the Stroke Symptoms

Recognizing the signs and symptoms of a stroke is essential for swift intervention to minimize the risk of damage to the brain. Understanding what to watch for before, during, and following a stroke can make all of the difference between having access to critical and swift medical attention or losing your life.

Before a Stroke

People who are more vulnerable to having a stroke might show indicators of danger or warning signs prior to the neurologic event. A lack of exercise, cigarette smoking, elevated cholesterol levels, and being overweight or obese are some of the associated hazards. Individuals may reduce their likelihood of having a fatal stroke by addressing these contributing factors, including modifications to their lives and regular visits to the doctor (WebMD, 2022).

In the Event of a Stroke

It's essential to identify the symptoms and indications of a cerebral infarction as promptly as possible. Unexpected numbness or weakness in a limb, arm, or face, particularly on one side, indicates the most widespread signs of stroke. Other signs could be trouble with vision, difficulty speaking or comprehending, abrupt disorientation, fainting, and severe headaches. If you or someone you care for suffers from these symptoms, you must seek medical help immediately (Maulden et al., 2005).

Neuroplasticity and Stroke

The human brain's incredible ability to reorganize and generate fresh connections between neurons, referred to as neuroplasticity, is essential for stroke recovery. When a cerebrovascular accident occurs, the cerebral cortex adapts and changes itself to compensate for the regions that were harmed. With therapy and recovery, this phenomenon allows patients to regain functions that have disappeared while improving their overall standard of life.

A knowledge of neuroplasticity concepts makes optimizing recovery results throughout rehabilitation following a stroke easier. Through targeted training sessions, treatments, and actions, individuals can use the brain's flexibility to promote ongoing recovery and allow functional improvements (Maulden et al., 2005).

Assembling Your Healthcare Team - Roles and Expectations

Managing the complicated nature of stroke recovery demands the support of a broad healthcare team dedicated to catering to the various needs of those affected by this neurological event. By recognizing vital members of the healthcare team and an in-depth understanding of their duties, you may work collaboratively to accomplish the best outcomes possible in ongoing medical treatment and recovery.

Identifying the Who and Why of Your Team

Rehabilitation Specialists - Why They Matter

Rehabilitation professionals are key players in the recovery procedure after a stroke. Experts such as physicians, occupational professionals, physiotherapists, speech and language pathologists, and neuropsychologists have the medical expertise to examine operational capacities, formulate customized rehab schedules, and enable you to regain your autonomy and reclaim your lost talents.

Doctors, with an emphasis on physical therapy and rehabilitation, or physicians, oversee patients through the whole rehabilitation process and coordinate care from various disciplines. Physical therapists use targeted workouts and psychological treatments to help clients gain greater power, equilibrium, and flexibility. Occupational therapy professionals help people regain their independence in everyday tasks like food preparation, cleaning, and clothes. These professionals treat stroke-related deficits in cognition, swallowing issues, and problems with communication. Neuropsychologists are responsible for cognitive capacities and treating mental health and cognitive issues.

By working closely with rehabilitation experts, stroke victims can access extensive and customized care aimed at optimizing functional recovery, improving quality of life, and encouraging reintegration into the community.

Long and Short-Term Monitoring

Stroke recovery is a continuing process that includes short- and long-term monitoring to assess progress, address emergent needs, and optimize results. Short-term monitoring involves regular assessments of vital signs, neurological status, and functional abilities during the acute phase of recovery, typically within the first few weeks following a stroke. Based on changing needs and therapy responses, these assessments inform decisions about immediate treatment and modifications to rehabilitation interventions.

Beyond the acute phase, ongoing surveillance includes regular assessments of mental, emotional, and physical well-being throughout the care spectrum. Healthcare providers may modify treatments to suit evolving demands while encouraging long-term healing and wellness by monitoring performance and acknowledging areas that require continuing difficulty or progress.

Navigating the System and Your Health

When patients start recovering from a stroke, they must understand what to expect and how to utilize the medical system successfully. By understanding the likely path of recuperation or the availability of supportive amenities, individuals may empower themselves to make intelligent choices and fight for what is best for them throughout the course of recovery.

What Does Recovery Look Like?

The method of healing after a stroke is highly customized and dynamic, and it is affected by an array of factors, including the nature and severity of the stroke, the efficacy of treatment and rehabilitation applications, and any existing underlying medical problems. While everybody recovers at various paces and to different extents, the path back to functioning and autonomy may have certain common themes and pivotal moments.

Stabilizing vital signs, minimizing problems, and starting rehabilitation efforts are of primary importance during the acute stage of recovery to reduce disability and optimize results. With prolonged therapy and medical oversight, people may see significant improvements in their speech, motor skills, and mental capacities throughout this period.

As the recovery process continues through the subacute and acute stages, the spotlight shifts to ongoing therapy and maintenance. In the long run, recovery from a stroke is an endeavor that requires resiliency, determination, and commitment to the achievement of important goals. By embracing an anticipatory mentality, participating in recovery endeavors, and employing relevant assistance and guidance structures, people can realize their highest potential and reestablish independence and general happiness after surviving a stroke (Maulden et al., 2005).

Useful Resources to Consider

Navigating the complexities of stroke recovery often requires access to a range of supportive resources and services. Consider the following resources to enhance your journey toward recovery:

- **Stroke support groups:** Participating in groups that cater to the emotional and physical needs of stroke victims offers possibilities of connecting and engaging with various stroke sufferers, exchanging narratives, and finding help and encouragement from colleagues.

- **Rehabilitation facilities:** Find respectable outpatient treatment or rehabilitation facilities that offer a wide range of treatments, such as vocational therapy, speech-language therapy, and physical therapy, that are suitable for fulfilling the needs of stroke victims.

- **Teaching resources:** For more information on strokes, treatment techniques, and local resources, read the internet pages, publications, and educational resources offered by respected institutions such as the Brain Foundation, National Stroke Association, and American Stroke Association. These groups will help you sustain the recovery process after a stroke.

- **Services of support for caregivers:** During the recuperation process, guardians have a vital role in supporting those who have experienced strokes. Analyze decisions for time off, training courses, and assistance services for caregivers, all of which aim to help and enhance the well-being of guardians.

By embracing these resources and leveraging the professionalism of healthcare workers, caregivers, and other survivors, stroke victims can successfully deal with the system, receive the assistance they desire, and walk the path to recovery while building resilience.

Emotional Resilience in the Face of Adversity

After a brain injury, treating the psychological consequences is vital in fostering an extensive recovery and general well-being. A wide range of challenges and mental anguish can be encountered by survivors of stroke and those near them as they handle the complexity of recovery and transitioning to life after the stroke.

What Types of Difficulties Are Possible?

- **Depression and anxiety:** Stroke survivors may experience feelings of despair or anxiety as a reaction to the unexpected shifts in their physical capabilities, autonomy, and standard of life. These emotional difficulties could be made worse by dementia, limitations in mobility, and unpredictability in the future.

- **Grief and loss:** Following a stroke, patients and their families may experience sorrow over lost skills, changed roles, and altered lifestyles. Getting used to occupational restrictions and depending on caretakers might be difficult for stroke survivors and their loved ones.

- **Fear and uncertainty:** Having a cerebrovascular accident may lead to worry and anxiety about upcoming medical problems, the potential of additional function loss, and the possibility of having a second stroke. Anxiety and stress could be exacerbated by concerns of being reliant, losing one's autonomy, and changing a person's character.

- **Social isolation:** Issues with communication, problems with mobility, and physical restrictions might affect interpersonal interactions and bring about loneliness and isolation. The inability of survivors of stroke to maintain social connections, take part in worthwhile activities, and get involved in community life could worsen psychological distress.

- **Coping with new realities:** Surviving a post-stroke existence means adjusting to fresh responsibilities, obstacles, and circumstances. The capacity for resilience, compassion for oneself, and confidence are essential for coping with shifts in one's perception of oneself, self-esteem, and feelings of loss of authority over how one lives.

Addressing the emotional impact of stroke requires a comprehensive approach that integrates psychological support, coping strategies, and social support networks. By acknowledging and validating the range of emotions experienced by stroke survivors and their caregivers, healthcare professionals can provide empathetic care and facilitate access to resources and interventions to promote emotional resilience and well-being.

Stress Management: Coping with the Recovery

Building mental strength after having a stroke is essential for conquering the difficulties of recovery and improving overall health. Stress management is vital to cope with the recuperation procedure's physical, emotional, and mental requirements.

- **Mindfulness and relaxation techniques:** Intensive breathing workouts, gradually implemented muscular relaxation, and meditation on mindfulness are proven ways to reduce stress while promoting relaxation. These daily habits can be integrated to improve coping abilities, reduce stress, and increase awareness of oneself (Maulden et al., 2005).

- **Creating a support system:** An extensive network of close friends, relatives, medical professionals, and support groups can provide social assistance, technical help, and psychological validation. Obtaining direction, discussing experiences, and finding help from peers can reduce thoughts of alienation and give a sense of togetherness.

- **Setting realistic goals:** Setting attainable goals and recognizing each minor accomplishment along the recuperation path can bolster your motivation, self-esteem, and feelings of achievement. Breaking down larger goals into feasible and measurable steps while aiming for progress more than perfection can lower feelings of overwhelm and increase confidence in one's ability to overcome challenges.

- **Indulging in meaningful activities:** Getting involved in pleasant, purposeful pursuits might bolster one's state of mind, lower one's anxiety, and improve mental health. Engaging in worthwhile pursuits, such as helping others, artistic endeavors, or interests, can provide meaning and direction and distract from the challenges of recovery.

- **Seeking professional support:** Psychiatrists or therapists, for instance, may provide personalized techniques for managing stress, controlling emotions, and building resilience. Personalized emotional control, capacity for problem-solving, and cognitive behavioral approaches could constitute the primary subjects during therapy sessions (Maulden et al., 2005).

- **Practicing self-care:** Self-care activities like obtaining sufficient rest, consuming a nutritious diet, exercising regularly, and investing in recreation time are crucial for managing stress and improving overall well-being. Having time to rest and take care of personal needs is also crucial for recovering from a stroke.

By incorporating these stress management techniques into their rehabilitation, patients may build mental toughness to cope with the challenges of cerebral therapy and enhance their general state of existence (Maulden et al., 2005). People can be encouraged to face each phase of rehabilitation with tenacity, courage, and perseverance by embracing a proactive mindset, seeking assistance whenever required, and placing a high value on taking care of themselves.

This chapter explored the complicated procedure of healing after a stroke, emphasizing the importance of mental fortitude in conquering rehabilitation difficulties and recovering a good quality of life. We first examined how a stroke could present itself and its psychological, mental, and bodily consequences. By learning about different kinds of strokes, assessing early warning signs, and understanding the opportunities for rehabilitation via neuroplasticity, you got a significant and knowledgeable look into your condition and potential for recovery and rehabilitation.

The creation of an effective and compassionate medical team that is ready to fulfill the unique needs of survivors of a stroke is vital to the healing process. Support systems, caregivers, and rehabilitation specialists play a crucial role in providing comprehensive therapy, promoting growth, and navigating the complicated workings of the medical system. By collaborating and sharing ideas, you can examine the support systems and resources required to maximize your recovery path and attain purposeful improvements in functionality and wellness. The next chapter discusses the critical relationship between nutrition and stroke.

NUTRITION AND STROKE

British scientists tell us that they have made a super broccoli that can assist in battling heart disease. If you want to defeat heart ailments, why don't you develop a meal people will certainly eat? Like a super glazed donut.

–Jay Leno

Food is essential for recovering from a stroke, given that it helps the human body's healing process, assists in recovery, and decreases the likelihood of future problems. A mantra from personal trainers is, "You can't out-train a bad diet." The same is true for your overall health. The bitter truth is that the vast majority of cases of chronic diseases such as stroke and heart disease are caused by lifestyle. The current standard American diet is full of processed and artificial foods that damage the endothelium, which is the inner lining of your blood vessels. When the endothelium is damaged, the end result is clogged arteries which causes heart disease, cerebrovascular disease, kidney disease, etc. The good news is that you have control over what you eat!

This part of the book will address which foods are particularly beneficial for stroke recovery. It will then look at the foods to completely shun, illustrating the bond between nutrition and wellness while recovering from a stroke.

The Connection Between Nutrition and Brain Health

A vital relationship exists between brain health and dietary tendencies, mainly concerning learning and memory. The best possible performance of your mind is directly affected by the substances you eat. Sustaining mental clarity while encouraging a healthy brain in general needs particular nutrients, including vitamins like B vitamins, which are present in vegetables and fruit, and fatty acids called omega-3, which are present in fish (Foroughi et al., 2013).

These vitamins and minerals are plentiful in a well-rounded diet that contributes to better memory, concentration, and ability to solve problems while reducing the risk of memory loss and illnesses, including Alzheimer's. On the other hand, eating a diet rich in sugar, refined foods, and saturated fats could harm mental abilities and increase the risk of brain decline. Knowing how food affects the brain's functioning emphasizes the importance of selecting nutritious foods to maintain cognitive energy throughout life.

Long-term Benefits of Eating Healthy

There are more long-term advantages to living healthily that transcend your physical health. What follows next are a number of the main benefits:

- **Decreased risk of chronic diseases:** A nutrition-rich diet full of vegetables, fruits, whole grains, lean protein, and good fats can all help avoid heart disease, type 2 diabetes, particular forms of cancer, and elevated blood pressure.

- **Better weight management:** A nutritious diet helps one maintain an appropriate weight, which is essential for overall health and decreases the possibility of contracting illnesses associated with being overweight (Foroughi et al., 2013).

- **Improved mood and mental health:** Eating foods with high amounts of nutrients benefits mental health and mood. Diets that include vegetables, fruit, appropriate grains, and fatty acids such as omega-3 have a core relationship with low depressive disorders and anxiety.

- **Improved cognitive function:** Consuming a nutritious diet full of antioxidants, minerals, and vitamins improves brain wellness and enhances mental skills, including memory, focus, and solving problems.

- **Stronger immune system:** Foods packed with micronutrients offer the immune system the antioxidants, vitamins, and minerals required to defend against illnesses and infections.

- **Better digestive health:** Consuming a recipe that contains whole vegetables, fruits, and grains filled with fiber improves the condition of the digestive tract while lowering the risk of significant problems, such as gas, diverticulitis, and constipation.

- **Longer lifespan:** Studies demonstrate that individuals who maintain a nutritious diet usually live longer and age better than those who fail to make healthy dietary choices (Foroughi et al., 2013).

- **Higher quality of life:** Over time, eating nutritiously may improve your energy levels, boost the quantity and quality of sleep you enjoy, and enhance your sense of all-around happiness, which may lead to an improved standard of life (Foroughi et al., 2013).

Making nutritious food a top concern may have a significant and lasting effect on your mental and physical health, contributing to a more joyful and fulfilling life.

Nutrients to Aid Stroke Recovery

Healing from a cerebral infarction is easily enhanced by eating a diet rich in vitamins and minerals, and the following nutrients are vital to this process:

- **Healthy fatty acids:** Omega-3 fatty acids are assumed to have anti-inflammatory qualities that might help lower swelling inside the brain after a stroke. They can be obtained in walnuts, the seeds of flax, and fatty fish such as mackerel, salmon, and sardines. These additionally encourage memory retention and neurological wellness (Foroughi et al., 2013).

- **Antioxidants:** Oxidative stress intensifies during a stroke and eventually damages cells. Antioxidant compounds, such as vitamins C and E, and the pigment beta-carotene, are present in large amounts in fruits, vegetables, nuts, and seeds. They might assist in the repair and redevelopment of damaged brain tissue.

- **Proteins:** Reconstructing broken cells and reclaiming muscle power are essential for stroke recovery. High-protein foods such as lentils, beans, soy, poultry, and fish are abundant in amino acids needed for tissue regeneration and repair.

Eating these essential nutrients may help physical and mental recovery after a stroke, decreasing the likelihood of future health issues. During recovery from a stroke, it is crucial to speak with a medical professional or an experienced dietitian to develop an individualized dietary strategy centered on food habits and unique needs.

Healthy and Unhealthy Foods to Consider

When thinking about ideal foods during stroke recovery, focusing on nutrient-dense selections that promote quick healing and general wellness while avoiding processed foods you consume is vital. Also, avoid foods high in unhealthy fats and sugars. Going through the following few examples will be critical for you:

Healthy Foods

- **Greens and fruits:** Loaded with antioxidants and vitamins, these foods encourage general health while giving essential minerals for recovery.

- **Whole grains:** High in nutrition and providing an uninterrupted power boost, whole grain foods, including brown rice, quinoa, and oats, additionally encourage healthy stool production and digestion.

- **Lean proteins:** Lentils, beans, tofu, poultry, and fish are good sources of lean proteins for building muscles and regenerating tissue.

- **Healthy fats:** Foods that contain beneficial fats, such as avocados, nuts, seeds, and olive oil, can provide essential fatty acids that encourage mental health and reduce inflammation.

- **Water:** Drinking sufficient water is necessary for optimal well-being and assists with movement, absorption, and mental alertness.

Unhealthy Foods

- **Processed foods:** Eating a lot of sodium, unhealthy fats, and artificial ingredients may hinder recovery and promote irritation. A good rule of thumb is that if you can't pronounce the ingredients, you shouldn't eat them. The recommendation is to eat most of your foods from Levels 1 and 2, avoid Level 3 and especially stay away from Level 4 foods. The Nova classification divides foods into four classes:

  - Level 1: unprocessed. Example: an apple
  - Level 2: processed culinary ingredients. Example: unsweetened applesauce
  - Level 3: processed foods. Example: apple pie
  - Level 4: ultra-processed foods, usually containing high fructose corn syrup. Example: apple pie from a fast food restaurant

- **Trans fats:** Fried items, prepackaged meals, and baked products are a few examples of foodstuffs that include trans fats, which may exacerbate inflammation and raise the risk of coronary artery disease and stroke.

- **Excess salt:** Items high in sodium chloride, such as tinned meals, processed meat, and junk food, may increase blood pressure levels and induce fluid retention, both of which may worsen the effects of a stroke.

- **Sugary beverages:** Sweet drinks, including fruit juices, energy drinks, sports drinks, and cola, have no nutritional value and may increase the level of sugar in your blood, which may be harmful to your overall health and recovery from a stroke.

- **Alcohol:** It's essential to limit drinking alcohol throughout the healing process in the aftermath of a stroke since it may interfere with medications, increase the likelihood of hemorrhaging, and decrease mental abilities (Foroughi et al., 2013).

Following a stroke, prioritizing nutritious meals and eliminating artificial and highly processed foods can speed up recovery while improving overall wellness.

Staying Hydrated

Maintaining good well-being and mental clarity demands adequate hydration. Since the human brain comprises approximately 75% fluid, even minor dehydration may enormously affect how one feels and thinks. Avoiding consuming sufficient amounts of water may result in several problems, such as:

- **Cognitive impairment:** Memory, also known as the ability to focus and remember while making choices, can easily be impacted by dehydration. Research has shown mild dehydration can harm clear cognition (National Council on Aging, 2021).

- **Mood shifts:** A parched body may experience changes in mood, irritability, and high stress levels. Staying adequately hydrated is essential for maintaining mental equilibrium and happiness (National Council on Aging, 2021).

- **Headaches:** Dehydration affects blood flow, including oxygen delivery to the mind, and may result in migraines and headaches.

- **Fatigue:** Poor hydration may lead to feeling tired with no or low energy, making it harder to concentrate and perform chores (National Council on Aging, 2021).

The relationship between the cerebral cortex and water highlights the importance of appropriate hydration for maximum cognitive performance and general well-being. The recommended number of fluids you should drink to be hydrated differs depending on your age, gender, amount of physical activity, the environment, and your overall well-being. While eight 8-oz glasses of fluids daily are usually suggested, individual requirements might vary (National Council on Aging, 2021). Specific individuals may need more fluids than others, such as those who reside in regions with high temperatures or engage in intensive sporting activities. A general guideline is to keep your urine a pale yellow color. And yes, that means you should look!

Why Does Hydration Matter?

There are many explanations for the reason why water is essential, particularly for the functioning of the brain:

- **Preserves fluid balance:** Consuming liquids aids in the ongoing maintenance of the body's fluid equilibrium, ensuring enough water for the body's tissues and cells. This equilibrium is needed for the mind to function at its peak and for overall wellness (National Council on Aging, 2021).

- **Improves nutrient transport:** Fresh water is required to eliminate waste products and poisons from the human body and deliver oxygen and vitamins to the brain. Keeping enough water enables nutrients to reach neurons more efficiently, maintaining their functioning and health.

- **Controls body temperature:** Water assists the body in eliminating heat via sweat, which controls body temperature. Staying hydrated helps prevent excessive heat, which may lead to pain and fatigue and hinder brain function (National Council on Aging, 2021).

- **Supports brain structure:** Because water occupies almost all of the cerebral cortex, staying hydrated is critical for maintaining the brain's sanity and framework. Dehydration may interfere with neural conjunction and cause brain cells to contract, which can harm cognition.

- **Improves cognitive performance:** Consuming fluids ensures the mind gets enough circulation and oxygen, improving memory retention. Drinking sufficient amounts of water also helps retain information, concentrate, and make decisions, which improves the brain as an entire system (National Council on Aging, 2021).

Proper hydration is essential for optimal cognition and health. Consuming sufficient fluids may help preserve the right amount of fluid, aid nutritional delivery, maintain the internal temperature, sustain the brain's structure, and increase mental abilities. Making water a top concern may promote beneficial brain wellness and overall health.

Drink More Fluids

- **Water:** Because it refreshes the human body without contributing carbohydrates or glucose, drinking water is vital for staying hydrated. It assists in maintaining fluid equilibrium and promotes all of the body's operations, particularly the workings of the mind (National Council on Aging, 2021).

- **Herbal Tea:** Besides keeping you well-hydrated, herbal beverages such as chamomile, peppermint, green or ginger tea offer additional health benefits. Their high level of antioxidants may help reduce irritation and increase resilience.

- **Coconut Water:** Abundant in potassium and other electrolytes, coconut water assists in recovering levels of minerals depleted through sweating. It is additionally inherently nourishing and is a calorie-efficient and pleasing alternative to sweetened sports beverages (National Council on Aging, 2021).

- **Vegetable Juice:** Juices made directly from vegetables, like beet, carrot, or lettuce, provide water and are an excellent supply of nutrients, vitamins, and minerals important for good heart health. They provide a nutrient boost while contributing to overall hydration.

Fluids to Minimize Consumption

- **Sweet Drinks:** Sugary beverages, such as cola, fruit juice, and vitality drinks, have higher added glucose content, and this can result in weight gain, dental decay, and ongoing illnesses such as obesity and heart disease.

- **Alcohol:** Drinking alcohol may dehydrate the body and disrupt mental operation. Also, too much alcohol can trigger thirst, fluid imbalances, and liver destruction. Consequently, it's necessary to ingest alcoholic beverages with caution and retain moisture via drinking water.

Those capable of supporting ideal hydration and general health by giving precedence to replenishing liquids such as water, herbal teas, coconut water, and plant-based juices. On the other hand, ingesting fewer sweet drinks and alcohol avoids too much sugar consumption and dehydration; this can contribute to better health results.

Role of Nutrition in Stroke Recovery

Food has an important effect on stroke recovery and is crucial to the whole rehabilitation process. The following are a few reasons why nutrition should be vital to the recovery plan.

Using Food for Stroke Recovery

A variety of variables need to be carefully taken into consideration when incorporating food into stroke recuperation:

- **Density of nutrients:** Choose a dietary regimen that contains nutrients, including meals rich in minerals, antioxidants, and vitamins, to help repair and promote good health. Pay attention to whole grains, vegetables, fruits, lean meat, and good fats (Foroughi et al., 2013).

- **Hydration:** Ingest a lot of fluids during the day to ensure proper hydration. Dehydration can increase stroke-associated complications, so remaining hydrated is vital for complete recovery.

- **Balanced diet:** Adopt a stable diet that consists of several food groups to give you all the essential nutrients for recovery. Add a mix of healthy fats, carbohydrates, and lean proteins to every meal to improve energy levels and repair brain cells.

- **Individual needs:** When planning a meal, consider dietary requirements, social norms, and dietary restrictions or intolerances. Adapt your diet depending on your specific needs and preferences, guaranteeing that recovery-critical micronutrients enter the body.

- **Meal Timing:** Pay attention to the sequence and separation of your dietary intake for better digestion and peak energy. More frequent, smaller meals spaced out during the day might benefit those with inconsistent appetites or digestion problems.

Select appropriate nutrients and quantities and collaborate with healthcare professionals for better healing and general well-being. People with restricted diets may continue to eat properly and support their recovery from a stroke by carefully evaluating their particular dietary desires and requirements, implementing needed changes, and collaborating with medical professionals to aid their recovery.

Impact of Sodium

Moderate consumption of sodium is suggested for an array of explanations:

- **Control of Blood Pressure:** Eating a lot of sodium raises blood pressure, which increases the probability of arterial hypertension, heart attack, stroke, and damage to the kidneys.

- **Fluid Balance:** Salt controls the human body's fluid balance. Too much salt may lead to edema, inflammation, and fluid retention, particularly in people with heart or kidney disorders.

- **Cardiovascular Health:** Eating a lot of sodium in your diet has been scientifically associated with an increased likelihood of suffering from cardiovascular diseases, including heart failure, cerebrovascular accidents, and strokes. Lowering sodium intake may decrease the possibility of some diseases and help enhance the cardiovascular system.

- **Kidney Function:** Eating excessive salt gradually causes your kidneys to get overworked and compromised, increasing the likelihood of kidney disease and heart failure.

Commonly Eaten Foods High in Sodium and Alternatives

- **Processed Meats (e.g., bacon, sausage, deli meats):** These food items are frequently high in added salt and chemical preservatives. Think about alternatives like fresh poultry, seafood, or lean cuts of meat with no added salt. Choose homemade sandwiches with newly cooked or barbecued meat instead of deli meats.

- **Canned Soups and Broths:** Canned soups, broths, and sauces often contain salt added to improve taste and sustain shelf life. Look for low-sodium or sodium-free varieties when you go shopping, or make your own homemade soups using fresh greens and broth with no added salt.

- **Processed snack foods:** Chips, pretzels, and crackers can be substantial sources of sodium because they frequently have a lot of added salt. Choose low-salted or unsalted varieties or healthier snacks like air-popped popcorn, fresh fruit, and vegetables.

- **Condiments and sauces:** Many sauces and condiments, such as soy sauce, ketchup, and salad dressings, are manufactured with high sodium content to increase flavor. Rather than adding more salt to dressings and sauces, try to find sodium-free or reduced-sodium options or make your own at home with vinegar, herbs, and spices.

One way for people to manage their salt intake and promote improved general health, especially kidney and cardiovascular health, is to avoid processed foods altogether or at least choose lower-sodium alternatives to high-sodium foods.

Examples of Diet Plans

Dietary Plan 1: Mediterranean Diet

- **Breakfast:** Avocado toast with nutritious grains and a dollop of Greek yogurt with fresh berries and almonds for breakfast.

- **Snack:** Dress a mixed green salad with vinegar and olive oil, then add grilled salmon, quinoa, and roasted veggies.

- **Lunch:** Consume carrots, cucumbers, and bell peppers cut with hummus.

- **Dinner:** The menu includes a Greek salad topped with feta cheese and olives, Mediterranean chicken skewers served with grilled vegetables, and whole grain couscous.

- **Benefits:** Nutrients such as lean proteins (like fish and poultry), whole grains, nuts, seeds, and healthy fats (like olive oil) are all abundant in the Mediterranean diet, which is rich in vitamins, minerals, antioxidants, and omega-3 fatty acids. The diet supports heart health, brain function, and general well-being. It may also lower the risk of chronic diseases, including heart disease and stroke.

Dietary Plan 2: Plant-Based Diet

- **Breakfast:** This meal consists of overnight oats based on almond milk, garnished with sliced bananas, almonds, and honey.

- **Lunch:** Try eating brown rice, chickpeas, and vegetable stir-fry. Also, eat mixed green salad dressed with balsamic vinaigrette.

- **Snack:** A fresh fruit salad topped with a few mixed almonds.

- **Dinner**: Steamed broccoli, roasted sweet potatoes, and a stew of lentils and vegetables.

- **Benefits:** A plant-based diet eliminates animal products while emphasizing entire, minimally processed plant foods, like fruits, vegetables, legumes, nuts, seeds, and whole grains. This diet is low in cholesterol and saturated fat and high in antioxidants, fiber, vitamins, and minerals. It is linked to many health advantages, including a decreased risk of heart disease, type 2 diabetes, obesity, and malignancies, as well as enhanced general health and longer life spans.

Using Dietary Professionals

People can seek advice from different kinds of dietitians based on their individual needs and objectives when it comes to meal planning. Typical food specialists to take into account are:

- **Registered Dieticians (RDs or RDNS) or registered nutritionists:** Experts in nutrition and dietetics, registered dietitians are qualified and licensed medical professionals. They offer customized meal plans, personalized nutrition counseling, and advice on handling certain medical conditions, such as heart ailments, diabetes, stroke, and weight control. RDs and RDNs can address dietary limitations, intolerances, and allergies and offer evidence-based recommendations for maximizing nutrition and general health.

- **Certified Nutrition Specialist (CNS):** CNSs are professionals with a certification in nutrition science who have completed extensive coursework and training. They create customized nutrition regimens, provide illness prevention, sports nutrition, and weight management, among other health objectives, and provide nutrition education and counseling.

- **Nutritionist:** Although there are no regulations governing the name "nutritionist" as there are for "dietitian," some nutritionists may hold degrees in nutrition science or related subjects and provide nutrition advice and counseling. A nutritionist's degree of training and experience can differ, so it's important to confirm their credentials and qualifications before using their services.

A licensed dietitian or other nutrition specialist can generally guarantee that people receive precise, scientifically supported dietary advice and support catered to their particular needs, preferences, and health objectives. These professionals can assist people with navigating dietary adjustments, optimizing nutrition for recovery, and implementing sustainable lifestyle changes to promote general health and well-being.

In Chapter 3, we learned that food is critical during the process of stroke recovery, impacting both physical and mental recovery. A nutritious diet abundant in lean proteins, vegetables, fruits, whole grains, and good fats offers key nutrients that help repair damaged brain cells, muscle vitality, and general healing after a stroke. It is also noted that adding anti-inflammatory meals, like those rich in omega-3 fatty acids and antioxidants, can assist in lowering irritation, improving brain wellness, and reducing secondary complications. By prioritizing hydration and reducing the consumption of salt while making informed food selections, you can maximize your nutrition to enable recovery and enhance long-term results after a stroke.

Finding proper assistance from food experts, like qualified dietitians or diet specialists, can offer significant help and individualized recommendations for implementing dietary changes and furthering maximum health during stroke recovery. These experts can provide customized meal plans, food education, behavior alteration tactics, and ongoing assistance to educate you to make life-long lifestyle changes that help your path to recovery. By tapping into the power of food, you can improve your physical and mental rehabilitation, lower the risk of complications, and increase your general quality of life after surviving a stroke.

Integrating Neuroplasticity and Diet

Neuroplasticity is the brain's ability to adapt its shape and function in response to mental experiences and activities.

–Norman Doidge

Chapter 4 explores the fascinating interaction between nutrition and neuroplasticity and its significant consequences for stroke recovery. As Norman Doidge explains, neuroplasticity allows the brain to rearrange and adapt to various stimuli, including dietary considerations. To provide insight into the possibility of nutritional components reducing the effects of stroke, this chapter examines how they exert control over neuroplasticity pathways.

Through a synthesis of research and clinical experiences, you will discover diet's critical role in supporting neuroplasticity after a stroke, enabling improved neuronal reconfiguration, functional recovery, and cognitive rehabilitation. This chapter provides hope for improving nutritional therapies to build resilience and accelerate recovery in stroke survivors by clarifying the complex relationships between nutrition and neuroplasticity.

Exploring the Synergy Between Neuroplasticity and Our Diet

Understanding the relationship between neuroplasticity and nutrition is essential to improving general mental health and brain function. The brain's extraordinary capacity to adjust and rearrange itself in response to experiences and environmental changes is known as neuroplasticity. Since diet supplies the nutrients required for brain health and function, it significantly impacts how neuroplasticity is shaped. Neurotransmitter production, neuroinflammation, and synaptic plasticity are all basic mechanisms that underpin neuroplasticity.

Nutrients like omega-3 fatty acids, antioxidants, vitamins, and minerals affect these processes. By understanding the synergy between neuroplasticity and food, we can apply dietary practices to maintain brain health, improve learning and memory, and even reduce the risk of neurological illnesses. This connection underscores the importance of adopting a nutritious diet as a critical component of maintaining optimal brain function throughout life (Psychology, 2021).

Optimizing brain health and cognitive performance requires understanding how nutrients affect neuroplasticity recovery. Neuroplasticity processes are supported by several essential nutrients, including:

- **Fish Oils (Omega-3):** The brain's neuroplasticity and overall health depend heavily on omega-3 fatty acids, especially EPA (eicosatetraenoic acid) and DHA (docosahexaenoic acid). These fatty acids facilitate synaptic transmission and function and are essential parts of the membranes of neurons. Furthermore, the anti-inflammatory qualities of omega-3 fatty acids can aid in reducing neuroinflammation and enhancing neuroplasticity regeneration. Omega-3 fatty acid-rich foods include walnuts, flaxseeds, chia seeds, and fatty fish (salmon, mackerel, and sardines) (Lin et al., 2018).

- **Antioxidants:** Antioxidants are chemicals that assist in scavenging dangerous free radicals, which can cause neurodegeneration and hinder neuroplasticity in brain tissue. By lowering oxidative stress, antioxidants promote synaptic plasticity, cognitive function, and neuronal survival. Vitamins C, E, beta-carotene, and flavonoids are a few examples of antioxidants. Berries, citrus fruits, leafy greens, and bell peppers are just a few examples of vibrant fruits and vegetables full of these chemicals (Psychology, 2021).

- **Amino Acids and Protein:** Protein is necessary for creating neurotransmitters, which are chemical messengers that help neurons communicate. Amino acids are essential for the synthesis of neurotransmitters and the flexibility of synapses. They are present in proteins. One neurotransmitter involved in mood regulation and cognitive function is serotonin, derived from the amino acid tryptophan (Lin et al., 2018).

- **Micronutrients:** The body requires essential minerals to sustain optimal health and function. They contain minerals and vitamins, iron, zinc, calcium, and vitamins A, C, D, E, and K. To maintain bone health, immunological response, metabolism, and other physiological functions, micronutrients are essential. Compared to macronutrients like proteins, lipids, and carbs, they are required in lesser amounts, but a shortage can have serious adverse effects on health (Lin et al., 2018). Thus, general health must maintain a balanced diet high in micronutrients.

By assuring sufficient consumption of these nutrients, people can facilitate the recovery of neuroplasticity, improve brain function, and foster general cognitive health.

Mindful Eating

Eating with awareness requires being present and focused on the process. Here are some tips to consider and reasons to give it a try:

- **Savor your food:** You can get the most out of your food by paying attention to its flavor, texture, and scent as you consume.

- **Better digestion:** Eating mindfully enables your body to detect signals of hunger and fullness more accurately, which can help promote healthy digestion.

- **Improved portion control:** Monitoring your body's hunger signals and fullness can help you avoid overindulging and foster a positive connection with food. Abandon your membership in the Clean Plate Club.

- **Decreased tension:** When eating mindfully, focusing on the present rather than ruminating about the past or the future might help reduce tension and anxiety (Psychology, 2021).

Incorporating these techniques into your daily routine can help you develop a healthier and more mindful relationship with food (Psychology, 2021).

Physical Exercises to Promote Neuroplasticity

Neuroplasticity refers to the brain's ability to reorganize itself by forming new neural connections throughout life. Physical activity promotes neuroplasticity by stimulating the brain to create these new connections. Exercise enhances blood flow to the brain, increases the production of neurotransmitters, and encourages the release of growth factors, all of which support neuronal growth and connectivity.

- **Aerobic exercises:** Running, cycling, swimming, and brisk walking increase blood flow to the brain, delivering oxygen and nutrients essential for neuronal health.

- **Strength training:** Resistance exercises like weightlifting stimulate the release of growth factors, which support the growth and repair of neurons.

- **Balance and coordination exercises:** Activities like yoga, tai chi, and balance training challenge the brain to adapt and coordinate movements, promoting neuroplasticity (Psychology, 2021).

Cognitive Exercises to Promote Neuroplasticity

The upcoming exercises improve neuroplasticity:

- **Learning new skills:** Activities such as playing a musical instrument, learning a new language, or mastering a new hobby stimulate the brain to form new connections and pathways.

- **Memory exercises:** Practicing memory games, puzzles, and tasks that require mental calculation or strategic planning can enhance cognitive function and promote neuroplasticity.

- **Mindfulness and meditation:** These practices have been shown to increase gray matter density in areas of the brain associated with memory, learning, and emotional regulation, promoting neuroplasticity (Psychology, 2021).

Importance of Diet and Exercise in Neuroplasticity

The link between diet and movement in neuroplasticity recovery is also significant. A healthy diet provides the nutrients necessary for brain function and repair, while movement enhances the body's ability to absorb and utilize these nutrients. Key dietary factors that support neuroplasticity include omega-3 fatty acids, antioxidants, vitamins, and minerals found in fruits, vegetables, whole grains, and lean proteins. Combining a nutritious diet with regular physical activity can optimize neuroplasticity recovery and promote overall brain health (Lin et al., 2018).

Factors Hindering Adherence to a Neuroplastic Diet

Several challenges can hinder adherence to a neuroplastic diet, impacting neuroplasticity and overall brain health:

- **Accessibility and affordability:** Healthy foods such as fresh fruits, vegetables, and fish can be expensive or inaccessible in some areas, making it challenging for individuals with limited resources to maintain a neuroplastic diet.

- **Cultural and social factors:** Dietary habits are often deeply ingrained within cultural and social contexts. Adopting a neuroplastic diet may clash with cultural food preferences or social norms, leading to resistance or difficulty making dietary changes.

- **Time constraints:** Busy lifestyles and hectic schedules can make prioritizing meal planning, cooking, and consuming nutrient-rich foods difficult. Fast food and processed options may seem more convenient, but they often lack the essential nutrients for brain health.

- **Food preferences and aversions:** Individuals may have specific tastes, preferences, or aversions that make it challenging to incorporate neuroplastic-friendly foods into their diet. For example, some people may dislike the taste or texture of certain vegetables or fish, limiting their options for neuroplasticity-promoting foods.

- **Marketing and misinformation:** Misleading marketing tactics and conflicting nutritional information can confuse consumers and make it challenging to discern which foods truly support brain health. Additionally, processed foods marketed as "brain-boosting" may contain additives and preservatives detrimental to neuroplasticity (Psychology, 2021).

- **Emotional and psychological factors:** Emotional eating, stress, depression, and other mental health issues can significantly impact dietary choices. Individuals may turn to comfort foods high in sugar, fat, and processed ingredients, which can hinder neuroplasticity and exacerbate cognitive decline.

Addressing these obstacles requires a multifaceted approach, including education, access to affordable healthy foods, support networks, and strategies to manage time and stress. Encouraging individuals to gradually introduce neuroplasticity-promoting foods into their diet, experimenting with new recipes and flavors, and seeking professional guidance from nutritionists or dietitians can help overcome these challenges and support long-term adherence to a neuroplastic diet.

Neuroplastic Eating Recommendations

To support neuroplasticity through diet, consider incorporating the following recommendations:

- **Omega-3 fatty acids:** Include sources of omega-3 fatty acids such as fatty fish (salmon, mackerel, sardines), flaxseeds, chia seeds, walnuts, and hemp seeds. These essential fatty acids support brain structure and function, promoting neuroplasticity (Lin et al., 2018).

- **Antioxidant-rich foods:** Consume a variety of fruits and vegetables high in antioxidants, such as berries (blueberries, strawberries, raspberries), dark leafy greens (spinach, kale), and colorful vegetables (carrots, bell peppers, tomatoes). Antioxidants protect the brain from oxidative stress and inflammation, supporting neuroplasticity.

- **Whole grains:** Choose whole grains like oats, quinoa, brown rice, and whole wheat bread over refined grains. Whole grains provide a steady supply of energy to the brain and contain nutrients like vitamin E, which supports cognitive function and neuroplasticity.

- **Lean proteins:** Add lean protein sources such as poultry, eggs, tofu, beans, and lentils to your meals. Protein is essential to neurotransmitter synthesis and repair of brain cells, facilitating neuroplasticity.

- **Healthy fats:** Incorporate sources of healthy fats such as avocados, olive oil, nuts, and seeds into your diet. These fats provide energy to the brain and support the production of neurotransmitters, promoting neuroplasticity.

- **Avoid processed foods:** Minimize the consumption of processed and ultra-processed foods high in refined sugars, unhealthy fats, and chemical additives. These foods can impair cognitive function and hinder neuroplasticity.

- **Stay hydrated:** Drink plenty of water throughout the day to maintain optimal brain function and support neuroplasticity. Dehydration can negatively impact cognitive performance and brain health.

- **Moderate alcohol consumption:** Limit alcohol intake to moderate levels, as excessive alcohol consumption can impair cognitive function and hinder neuroplasticity.

- **Mindful eating:** Practice mindful eating by paying attention to hunger and fullness cues, savoring each bite, and being aware of the sensory experience of eating. Mindful eating can help regulate appetite, reduce stress-related eating, and support overall brain health.

- **Herbs and spices:** When you cook, use herbs and spices with neuroprotective properties, such as turmeric, ginger, cinnamon, and rosemary. These herbs and spices contain compounds that have been shown to reduce inflammation, enhance cognitive function, and support neuroplasticity. Adding them to your meals can boost flavor and provide added brain health benefits.

Incorporating these neuroplasticity-friendly foods and habits into your diet can nourish your brain, support cognitive function, and promote neuroplasticity for optimal brain health and performance (Psychology, 2021).

In Chapter 4, we explored the vital role of diet in promoting neuroplasticity and supporting brain health. Individuals can nourish their brains and enhance their cognitive function by incorporating nutrient-rich foods and mindful eating practices. Overcoming obstacles, such as accessibility and cultural factors, is essential for maintaining adherence to a neuroplastic diet, empowering individuals to take control of their brain health. Moving forward into Chapter 5, we will explore physical rehabilitation strategies that complement neuroplasticity-promoting diets. Physical rehabilitation facilitates neuroplasticity and promotes recovery from neurological conditions, from aerobic exercises and strength training to balance and coordination activities. Individuals can optimize their brain's ability to adapt and thrive by integrating diet and physical rehabilitation strategies, fostering resilience and vitality throughout life.

Physical Rehabilitation Strategies

Not rest, but activity and therapy, heal the heart best.
                                                                    –Joerg Teichmann

The above quote is a powerful weapon to lay the groundwork for a revolution-like recovery method. To empower you with knowledge of physical rehabilitation strategies, this chapter will introduce you to goal-setting skills required to navigate life post-stroke, physiotherapy techniques necessary to improve mobility, and occupational therapy exercises to sustain your recovery.

Goal Setting Post Stroke

Adequate goal setting is a pivotal part of rehabilitation following a stroke, and it needs to be done carefully. Being realistic is crucial while making goals after a stroke, considering the overall status of the individual, including the level of functioning, risk factors, and safety concerns. Goals should focus on safety the most since this includes the possibility of injuries or misalignments during the recovery and rehabilitation journey (Lee et al., 2016).

It is essential to set goals after a stroke. Objectives should be devised so individual achievements will be recognized. The process will be gradual but not necessarily straight and can have occasional slips. Successive short-term goals that ultimately lead to more significant milestones enhance motivation and continuity of momentum throughout the rehabilitation process (O'Dell et al., 2009).

Physiotherapy Techniques for Strengthening and Mobility

Physical therapy, or physiotherapy, is a healthcare profession whose sole purpose is to use physical strategies, such as exercise, manual therapy, education, and other intervention modes, to restore and maintain mobility and well-being. In terms of stroke recovery, physiotherapy is of great importance because it allows patients affected by a stroke to improve their ability to move, muscle strength, and balance (O'Dell et al., 2009).

How Stroke Affects Physiotherapy

A person who suffers a stroke can have different types of physical problems, including muscle weakness, spasticity, balance failings, coordination failures, and also reduced mobility. Stroke survivors encounter not only physical deficits but also emotional and cognitive impairments. Physiotherapy aims to treat these conditions through specialized exercise programs, hands-on techniques, and functional training to help with walking, independence, and quality of life (O'Dell et al., 2009).

Why Physiotherapy Matters

Physiotherapy is important for the following reasons:

- **Improving mobility:** The main goal of physiotherapy is to enhance patients' movement capability, which, in turn, helps them live more independently and freely.

- **Enhancing strength and endurance:** Physiotherapy activities build strength and endurance, allowing stroke survivors to perform their daily life duties with less complication.

- **Restoring balance and coordination:** Physiotherapy interventions focus on restoring patients' balance and coordination, which helps decrease fall risk and increase overall stability (O'Dell et al., 2009).

- **Pain management:** A physiotherapy approach with massage and heat application can tackle the pain and sensation of discomfort produced from muscle stiffness, spasticity, or other special afflictions following a stroke.

- **Optimizing function:** Physiotherapy is a therapeutic method dedicated to improving body functions and peak performance in stroke patients. It makes recovery easier and has better long-term benefits.

Physiotherapy Exercise Regimens

Exercise programs facilitate getting back on track after a certain period of time.

Range of Motion Exercises

Form your own workouts, do them often, and challenge yourself. Examples include:

- **Neck rotations (sitting):** This is a single relaxation technique in which you gently turn your head to one side, hold for a couple of seconds, and then return to the center. Repeat on the other side. Do ten reps per side.

- **Shoulder rolls (standing):** Take your shoulders, bring them up to your ears, then circle them backward and down. Repeat for 15-20 repetitions (O'Dell et al., 2009).

- **Ankle circles (sitting or standing):** This involves rotating your feet in circles, first to the right and then to the left. Go for ten circles clockwise and counter-clockwise movement for each foot.

- **Knee extensions (sitting):** Extend one leg, hold for a while, and return to the starting position. Repeat with the other leg. Now, do ten on each leg and complete another two circuits.

- **Wrist flexion/extension (sitting):** Bring your hand up and down. Perform 15-20 wrist rotations each way.

- **Spine twists (sitting):** Sit upright and twist the torso first to one side and then to the other, returning to the center between the twists. Perform the following ten times, twisting on one side and then repeating on the other side.

What do Range of Motion Exercises and Recovery Have in Common

- **Maintain joint flexibility:** Flexibility, trained by the range of motion exercises, reduces the risk of stiffness and contractures and provides better mobility in general. It is beneficial in such a way for the joints as it contributes to keeping them flexible through these exercises (Lee et al., 2016).

- **Increase circulation:** These exercises, which engage the joints through the full range of motion, can elevate blood flow to the tissues near the joints, which in turn can help deliver nutrients and oxygen to the muscles and the joints themselves. The renewed flow of venous blood has the added benefit of removing waste products from the tissues, which, in turn, facilitates faster healing (O'Dell et al., 2009).

- **Prevent muscle weakness:** Range-of-motion exercises are the way to prevent muscle disengagement, which can be the effect of inactivity or an injury. Joints and muscles get strained when you perform the various activities of the day. Through range-of-motion exercises, you can keep your muscles strong and functional, thus maintaining easy mobility for proper movements.

- **Reduce pain and discomfort:** A range-of-motion workout accesses the area where pain/discomfort is present, which further helps deter or eliminate the issue at hand. Slowly putting joints and tissues through their full range of motions is believed to help reduce stiffness and enhance joint lubrication, thus promoting tissue regeneration that quickly reduces pain and improves overall comfort (Lee et al., 2016).

- **Enhance recovery:** Range of motion exercises have a variety of benefits in the recovery period. They enhance healing and restore function, and they help to avoid future problems like muscle loss or joint stiffening. These exercises are not only frequently a central part of physical therapy programs to guide individuals through injury, post-surgery, or chronic condition recovery but also to make significant contributions to overall health maintenance (O'Dell et al., 2009).

Strength Exercises

Strength exercises might help recovery in different ways depending on the exact condition you are suffering from. It is even possible to get some mental recovery at this stage. Here are four types of strength exercises, both sitting and standing and how they can help with recovery:

- **Bodyweight squats (standing):** Squatting with one's body weight immensely improves the muscles in the quadriceps, hamstrings, glutes, and core region. Increasing lower body strength can help with stability, balance, and functional ability, which are very important for many normal day-to-day activities like walking and rehabilitating from lower body injuries or surgeries.

- **Seated leg extensions (sitting):** When seated leg extensions are performed, the quadriceps muscles of the legs will work efficiently to stabilize and extend the leg. Refinement of these muscles helps stabilize the knee joint. Knee stability can be invaluable to individuals who have damage to their knee joints or have had knee surgery (O'Dell et al., 2009).

- **Standing calf raises (standing):** Calf raises develop the calf muscles, boosting ankle strength and stability. This activity has unique health benefits for those rehabilitating from ankle injuries and those looking to develop lower body strength and balance.

- **Seated rows (sitting):** Rowing concentrates on the upper back, shoulders, and arms when you process in a semi-seated position. Strengthening these muscles will not only help improve posture and shoulders but also can aid in increasing upper body strength. This may help individuals after upper body injuries or recovery from upper body surgeries (Lee et al., 2016).

Occupational Therapy Strategies for Daily Life Skills

Occupational therapy (OT) is an inclusive and multi-disciplinary healthcare approach whose central goal is to improve the participation of individuals of all age groups in purposeful occupations to improve their health, overall well-being, and independence. From the point of view of a therapist, they help patients with stroke recovery overcome the obstacles that stand in the way of performing their regular actions and achieving the independence they aim for (Lee et al., 2016).

Role of Occupational Therapy for Those Recovering from Physical Trauma

Occupational therapy helps you recover from physical trauma by enabling the following aspects:

- **Regaining independence:** Through occupational therapy, stroke survivors are taught to perform basic everyday tasks such as dressing, grooming, eating, and functional home activities to enable independence and improve the quality of life (Lee et al., 2016).

- **Improving motor skills:** Occupational therapy aids in the acquisition of fine motor skills, coordination, and balance while working for the above-mentioned purposes.

- **Enhancing cognitive abilities:** While physically helping patients regain the capabilities to move and intellectually assisting them with the development of skills required for performing daily activities such as memory, attention, problem-solving, and sequencing, occupational therapists equally ensure that these activities are undertaken effectively (Lee et al., 2016).

Environmental Adjustments or Modifications

Environmental adjustments or modifications are necessary to accommodate stroke survivors. Let's look at some of the recommended techniques that you can use.

Returning Home Considerations

When going back home after a stroke, think about the following:

- **Safety:** A stroke survivor must be conscious of safety measures, remove tripping hazards, use grip rails, and good lighting to avert falls and accidents (O'Dell et al., 2009).

- **Accessibility:** Adapt your home space to facilitate movement, for example, reorganizing furniture for pedestrians' convenience, installing ramps or stairlifts, and ensuring that the tools regularly used are available (Lee et al., 2016).

- **Support systems:** Establish a family support system with members, caregivers, or health professionals at home to provide what is necessary and applicable; encourage them throughout the process.

- **Routine and structure:** Creating a daily structured plan can empower stroke sufferers to put the scheduled activities, medications, physical therapy visits, and daily self-help requirements in order.

Possible Environmental Modifications

It is important to make the next set of modifications to an environment that will accommodate a stroke survivor:

- **Bathroom modifications:** Installing hand bars, non-slip mats, and a raised toilet seat to reduce slipping and increase safety in the bathroom (O'Dell et al., 2009).

- **Kitchen adaptations:** Counters can stabilize, and cooking utensils designed for adaptive use can be purchased or manufactured. In addition, kitchen items should be organized so that needed items are within reach to make meal preparation easier (Lee et al., 2016).

- **Bedroom adjustments:** Creating a quiet and secure sleeping area features a comfortable bed with quality bedding, any support pillows, and necessities at hand.

Through the implementation of these adaptations and modifications, stroke rehabilitation gives stroke survivors the ability to live in an environment that is supportive and safe with the purpose of the recovery process and feeling generally good.

Use of Speech and Language Therapy

The use of speech and language therapy in dealing with communication problems or issues is crucial to recovery from stroke. Let's turn our attention to some of the triggers of speech and language impairment after a stroke.

Causes of Speech and Language Impairment After a Stroke

Speech issues after a stroke are called aphasia and are due to damage to the language centers of the brain, particularly the left part of it. The two main areas of the brain responsible for language processing are:

- **Broca's area:** Broca's area is found in the frontal lobe, and the consequences of its impairment are connected with involuntary gestures in movement and speech articulation (Lee et al., 2016).

- **Wernicke's area:** In Wernicke's area, which is in the temporal lobe of the brain, we find the language processing and understanding centers. Damage to this area leads to difficulty in speech that makes sense and also can cause trouble with writing skills.

If the impact of a stroke is felt in these areas or where the connections between them are located, it may be possible to observe a couple of types of aphasia, impacting a person's ability to speak, understand language, read, and write (O'Dell et al., 2009).

How to Regain and Re-Establish Speech and Language

Speech and language exercises will help improve communication after suffering from a stroke. Below are some prescribed training methods:

Speech Exercises

- **Repetition exercises:** Practice pronouncing words and phrases, and then start reading sentences to improve articulation and fluency.

- **Articulation exercises:** Paying attention to clearly pronouncing sounds and syllables will help you enhance your speech.

- **Breathing exercises**: Work on respiration control and the mechanisms of voice support to increase vocal power and stamina.

- **Tongue and lip exercises:** Include tongue strengthening exercises in the program and better lip muscles for proper speech production.

- **Vocalization exercises:** Consider vocal drills, which will, in the long run, help build pitch, loudness, and tone in speech (Lee et al., 2016).

Language Exercises

- **Word retrieval exercises:** Work on labeling objects, activities, and topics to enhance the vocabulary function.

- **Phrase completion exercises:** Include simple sentences or sentence fragments in the speech to help learners improve their language production and grammar system.

- **Reading aloud:** Read the pieces or the whole passages out loud with a focus on the accuracy of pronunciation, fluency, and comprehension.

- **Picture description:** Present imaginary drawings or images to aid with developing speaking skills and increase your vocabulary.

Through systematized delivery of speech and language exercises, stroke survivors may stimulate the formation of new neural connections and yield positive effects on their language abilities. Consequently, they may improve their communication abilities. Speech-language pathologists and therapists will help the recovery process by improving speech skills and language ability during rehabilitation, another way individuals can achieve the objective (Lee et al., 2016).

Non-Traditional Therapies to Consider

The generic approaches to stroke recovery include medications, physical therapy, language therapy, and re-learning skills, as well as surgical or other invasive procedures for some patients. While the well-celebrated and effective modus operandi should be followed, alternative remedies offer even higher support. Here are five alternative therapies that can complement traditional approaches for stroke patients:

- **Acupuncture:** Acupuncture, on the other hand, refers to the placement of thin needles on pre-defined parts of the body, thereby healing and relieving some pain. It is recommended for stroke victims to normalize blood circulation, diminish muscle spasms, ease pain, and help cope with all of them.

- **Music Therapy:** Music therapy is a technique that uses music to satisfy different physical, psychological, cognitive, and social needs within a person. Music therapy can help stroke patients boost their motor skills, put them in a good spirit, lower stress and anxiety, and facilitate communication.

- **Yoga and Tai Chi:** These mind-body practice techniques require gentle exercises, breathing manipulation, and mindfulness sensation. Stroke patients can improve their balance and flexibility, strengthen their muscles, lessen stress, and improve their mental focus and emotional well-being.

- **Art Therapy:** Art therapy can simultaneously heal physical, mental, and emotional well-being. For stroke patients, it can be a wonderful method to improve their cognitive functions, create better self-expression, process emotions, and relieve stress.

- **Virtual Reality Therapy:** VR treatment in which the session participant experiences a real environment and activities through immersive methods. Virtual reality therapy for stroke patients can be used for rehabilitation by improving motor function, balance, coordination, and cognitive abilities in a motivating and engaging way.

How Alternative Therapies Can Benefit Stroke Patients

- **Diverse Treatment Options:** Apart from conventional methods, alternative therapies give stroke patients other options and a chance to experience more diverse treatments, with an add-on customized approach to recovery.

- **Reduced side effects:** Alternative therapies involve little to no side effects compared with some drugs and therapeutic interventions while presenting safer options for patients, especially those hypersensitized to traditional medications or medical procedures (Lee et al., 2016).

- **Improved quality of life:** Alternative therapies can help stroke patients improve their well-being. They encompass physical symptoms and emotional and psychological well-being, thus making this alternative a solid journey to healing and self-empowerment (O'Dell et al., 2009).

- **Long-term wellness:** Integrative medicine in stroke rehabilitation provides extra health care assistance, motivating patients to achieve optimum wellness, which includes but is not limited to the physical, mental, and emotional parts of the body. This allows patients to lead an enjoyable lifestyle after an illness (Lee et al., 2016).

Conventional treatments will surely continue to be a part of stroke treatment strategies and the road to complete recovery, but innovative and unconventional methods will also hold their own as they've been proven useful at some point. Collaborative work between health care providers and patients to assess and select a range of treatment options adds to a personalized and detailed plan to help stroke patients attain the best care.

Chapter 5 discussed the importance of establishing operational standards or physical goals in the recovery process since this contributes to the patient's recovery and well-being. Subsequently, by measuring realistic goals, individuals can begin their journey of physical rehabilitation.

Next, in Chapter 6, we will discuss cognitive rehabilitation strategies. We will acquire practical skills and competence in post-injury and impairment improvement in cognitive functions. Brain damage caused by an incident stops or disturbs the mind's working memory, attention, mental skills, and problem-solving. This part of the recovery affects the rehabilitation of the brain. Through providing structured cognitive exercises and ways, people can recover cognitive function as requested, take responsibility for their daily lives, and further their quality of life a step forward.

COGNITIVE REHABILITATION STRATEGIES

You can do the things you want to do, and you have the power to think about them positively or negatively. It is up to you, isn't it? At that very moment, you'll come to it and believe it.

–Marcus Aurelius

In this chapter, we alter our theme to cognitive rehabilitation methods, and we do so after Marcus Aurelius has put forward some enlightening and insightful words in the opening quotation. It reveals techniques that aid cognitive exercise, allowing people to regain mental strength and resistance. Chapter 6 explores the process, which emphasizes intrinsic processes instead of indicative cases, and surveys the role of mental performances, cognitive training, and adaptive strategy in manifesting themselves in positive cognitive activities.

Let's go on a path of self-exploration and empowering experiences in which you will learn how to manage your mind and use it to go beyond your beliefs about limits and excel in cognition. The body of this chapter aims to assure all those who are constant seekers of their cognitive welfare.

Rebuilding Memory Function Post-Stroke

Given the same conditions, a stroke can lead to impaired memory. The neural circuits responsible for these processes may be affected in the damaged region of the brain. The impact of a stroke on memory can manifest in various ways, including:

- **Short-term memory impairment:** Memory may be damaged entirely, leaving the individual unable to remember events soon after the stroke. This is a daunting hurdle since the power to remember is supposed to be the core function of your long-term memory (Mulhern, 2023).

- **Long-term memory difficulties:** Stroke survivors may experience an interruption in their memory and have difficulty retrieving information, facts, or previous events.

- **Confusion and disorientation:** Because of the cognitive consequences of a stroke, memory & organization of thoughts can be a challenge, from short to long-term memory interventions (Mulhern, 2023).

- **Difficulty with memory retrieval:** A stroke may leave the stroke survivor perplexed, as they might not recall even well-stored memories.

Interpreting memory impairment as one of the causes of a stroke is a mandatory step for working out efficient memory restoration strategies and the betterment of post-stroke cognitive function.

Memory Exercises

Memory training is crucial for sharpening mental function, better memory, and building a healthy mind. Here are five memory-focused exercises, along with how they help improve memory:

- **Memory games:** The mental activities required in memory games, like matching games, crossword puzzles, and sudoku, challenge the brain to recall information, rearrange and consolidate neural connections, and boost the pace of the brain's accuracy in thinking.

- **Mindfulness meditation:** Regular mindfulness meditation can heighten attention and focus and reduce stress levels. This will advance memory by encouraging relaxation, increasing brain flexibility, and improving cognitive ability.

- **Mnemonic devices:** Mnemonic devices, such as acronyms, visualization, or memory palaces, are one strategy for helping you organize and access information more easily.

- **Daily brain teasers:** Solving riddles, brain teasers, or logic puzzles can improve critical thinking skills, memory retention, and problem-solving abilities, resulting in optimal cognitive functions and memory.

- **Physical exercise:** Repetitive physical exercises, such as aerobics, may help augment blood flow to the brain, facilitate neurogenesis processes, and improve memory by enabling the brain to produce new brain cells and maintain high brain health levels.

- **Learning a new skill:** Skills-based activities, such as learning a new musical instrument, language, or hobby, can significantly grow the brain's plasticity through connecting new synapses, advanced memory retention, and increased cognitive function (Mulhern, 2023).

- **Chunking:** Chunking consists of breaking down the data into more understandable and manageable forms containing smaller pieces. The aim is to allow you to easily remember and recall complex details and sequences, which is done by arranging information in a meaningful way or grouping it together.

These exercises fortify memory by encouraging the brain to keep up with the challenge, to advance neuroplasticity while exposing the brain to new experiences, and to build stronger neural connections.

Memory Strategies

Strategies for memory retention are vital to improving memory capacity, sharpening the cognitive power of an individual, and, eventually, increasing productive learning. Proper memory techniques allow you to combine new information instead of just perceiving it as short-term memory and then storing it as long-term memory. This action will subsequently result in greater confidence and promptness when you need to recall those memories. The benefits of having good memory strategies include the following:

- **Improved retention:** These cognitive tactics empower you to encode and store information in your brain efficiently, thus improving your learning efficiency.

- **Enhanced recall:** This action is enhanced through the dance of memory strategies that can retrieve information from storage and enable memory recall and recognition.

- **Reduced forgetfulness:** Learning tips help you remember details and the relationship between topics better. This will improve your memory and automatically minimize forgetfulness.

- **Enhanced learning:** Learning to apply memory-enhancing methods in situations through education can help in understanding, picking up, and applying knowledge, therefore improving learning outcomes and the realization of effective academic performance (Mulhern, 2023).

By applying memory strategies while you execute daily tasks and undertake learning exercises and other cognitive functions, you can fully utilize the power of your memory. This helps create healthy cognitive function and strengthens mental performance in different aspects of life.

Improving Attention and Concentration

After going through the devastating effects of a stroke, attention span is negatively impacted, and no matter how hard you exercise patience, you may get distracted too easily. What you need to understand is that after suffering a stroke, your brain is damaged and fails to function effectively. The following are ways in which attention and concentration are affected:

- **Reduced focus:** Reduced focus impacts stroke survivors with problems maintaining concentration or getting involved in activities or conversations without being easily distracted. They are said to be experiencing a shortened attention span.

- **Difficulty with divided attention:** Stroke survivors may experience difficulties multitasking. This is because the brain gets overwhelmed when dividing attention between stimuli or tasks simultaneously, reducing performance and efficiency.

Exercises to Improve Attention - Focused Attention

Exercises that aim at focused attention can be helpful for people to improve their skills at concentrating on specific tasks or stimuli. Examples of exercises focused on attention include:

- **Deep breathing exercises:** Deep breathing methods can equip individuals to improve their attentiveness and concentration by bringing about calmness, stress reduction, and inner clarity (Mulhern, 2023).

- **Mindfulness meditation:** Mindfulness meditation exercises allow you to practice the art of focus and attention by helping the mind stay present in the current situation. This results in sharp concentration and cognitive work as your perception improves.

- **Visual tracking exercises:** Visuals that involve tracking the movements of objects in motion or following their moving patterns can be suitable activities that demonstrate focused attention. In this case, participants must concentrate selectively on specific visual stimuli and maintain focus for an extended period.

- **Listening exercises:** Implementing active listening workouts is very fruitful, such as listening to music or audiobooks that demand attention and concentration.

- **Memory games with a focus:** Some games, including concentration games or matching tasks, can help you focus. These games can help you sharpen your attention, enabling you to influence your cognitive processes when you play them positively.

These exercises are helpful tools for recovering attention and concentration after a stroke. They can improve cognition and help people return to their previous state and enjoy their lives again.

Selective Attention

For this book, we will describe selective attention as the capacity to pay attention precisely to significant stimuli while ignoring the unnecessary or distracting elements in the external environment (Mulhern, 2023).

Exercises for Selective Attention

- **Stroop test:** This practical exercise in cognitive psychology asks an individual to name the color of ink used in printing words, which is quite different from the words used. This test checks selective attention by highlighting the ink color and the ability to ignore the reaction after reading the prescribed section.

- **Selective listening tasks:** To improve your selective attention, take part in programs where you attentively listen to discourse while you pick out particular details, words, tones, or persons speaking.

- **Visual search exercises:** Practice visual search tasks where you must find special objects or patterns in congested pictures, training your skill to focus purposefully on important information amid distractions.

Divided Attention

Divided attention is the ability to direct your attention towards more than one task or stimuli that occurs almost simultaneously. It requires you to manage multiple task requirements on the go. After a stroke, divided attention may play an important role in individual recovery of cognitive functions. Cognitive training might improve the effectiveness of processing and the retention of information within stroke patients. The following are three exercises that focus on divided attention and can be beneficial for reconstructing memory function post-stroke:

- **Dual-task training:** This task involves combining two tasks with active participation, such as listening to a story and solving a crossword puzzle. By participating in two functional tasks that your mind focuses on, you can develop a strong and well-encapsulated skill in efficiently dividing your attention (Mulhern, 2023).

- **Multitasking activities:** Doing multiple tasks simultaneously, such as following a recipe while cooking, can help someone practice multiple attention splitting. These exercises offer several inputs to memory, which could be very helpful in its restoration since your brain needs to process and store information from multiple sources.

- **Simon Says:** It is important to do kindergarten-like activities that require a person to listen to a set of instructions and then perform all the actions correctly. In this case, your cognitive skills may improve since you must perform listening and executing tasks, wherein paying attention to one takes them away from the other.

How to Improve Concentration

It is vital to start by understanding the fundamental difference between concentration and attention.

Difference between Concentration and Attention

'Focusing' and 'concentration' are terms often used interchangeably but are only logically related expressions. The process of verbal communication includes focusing on a single stimulus or task, usually known as attention, while the main point of concentration is to keep the attention alive for some time. Attention is the first act of concentrating on anything in particular. At the same time, concentration, on the other hand, indicates the ability to keep the focus on it (Mulhern, 2023).

Ways to Improve Concentration

- **Mindfulness meditation:** When the mind is engaged during meditation, being mindful means staying present in the here and now. If practiced consistently, the brain eventually creates flexibility and strengthens attention. Performing meditation activities as a routine can improve your attention while neutralizing other thoughts before they interfere with your mind (Mulhern, 2023).

- **Break tasks into smaller activities:** Splitting complex tasks into smaller, more relevant, straightforward actions can help you develop flexibility in your approach and concentration. By focusing on completing one step at a time, you can avoid feeling overwhelmed and stay more engaged in the task at hand.

- **Limit distractions:** Watching your surroundings helps you focus and improve your concentration. This involves not logging in on your phone, avoiding distracting notifications, choosing a quiet workspace, and turning off anything distracting.

- **Practice regular exercise:** Research has demonstrated that physical exercise is vital for improving concentration. A daily routine of physical activity could improve blood flow to the brain, help boost mood, and contribute to concentration and attention (Mulhern, 2023).

- **Get sufficient sleep:** Good sleep and rest patterns enable the best cognitive processes, including concentration. Lack of sleep can lead to difficulty focusing and understanding; get at least 7 hours of sound sleep each night to help your brain function better. Taking naps is okay as long as they don't interfere with your nightly sleep. Also, non-sleep deep rest (NSDR), a term coined by neuroscientist Andrew Huberman, is a set of techniques for achieving deep relaxation and a restorative state without actually falling asleep.

Implementing these techniques in your daily routine can improve your attention span and enable you to live in the present. If you want to recover effectively from a stroke, use mindfulness to minimize interruptions. You can also keep yourself physically active and ensure you get much-needed sleep because all these factors contribute to the ability to concentrate and understand effectively (Mulhern, 2023).

Perception and Sensory Changes

- **Sensory:** Sensory is the process of getting information from the surrounding environment through sensory organs like the eyes, ears, skin, smell, and tongue. The sensory system is a tool that enables individuals to see, hear, feel, and react to the stimulation they receive. It is the precursor of perception.

- **Perception:** Perception is how people interpret the data from their environment. Sensory information is processed to be classified, specified, and assimilated to form a significant view of the universe.

Impairments in perception after stroke and changes in sensory function are well-known consequences.

Brain damage following a stroke may alter points of view and physiological function of sensory organs. Common effects include the reorganized processing of sensory details (extending to touch, vision, and hearing), modifications in spatial awareness, imbalances in body awareness (proprioception), and accurate interpretations of sensory information.

Sensory Integration Exercises

Sensory integration exercises, referred to as activities, are aimed at helping individuals subdue the task of processing and responding to sensory information efficiently. These games allow you to develop the faculties of vision and hearing in a way that you can use to process sensory input effectively. The end result is improved sensory processing. Here are three sensory integration exercises that can be beneficial post-stroke:

- **Proprioceptive activities**: Activities that provide deep pressure input, such as weightlifting or pushing against an opposing stimulus, can help one improve one's sense of body awareness and proprioception post-stroke (Mulhern, 2023).

- **Visual tracking exercises:** These activities include motion tracking and visual monitoring, such as looking at patterns with the eyes to enhance the visual processing and coordination of your body and mind.

- **Auditory discrimination tasks:** Active participation in activities that require discriminating among various noises or concentrating on a specific auditory cue enhances the auditory system's processing ability.

Adaptation Exercises

Adaptation exercises are important in rehabilitating a stroke patient's motor skills and cognitive abilities. They can be used to restore the functions that the patient lost and increase the quality of life. Doing this kind of exercise is supposed to help cope with new disabilities and may help to recover from a stroke. The focus here is to optimize the rehabilitation outcomes and quality of life. Here are five adaptation exercises that can be beneficial post-stroke:

- **Balance exercises:** A stroke can negatively impact balance. Exercises specifically for balance can help avert falls and make you more stable. Some examples are exercising on one leg, walking with your feet side by side, and weight-shifting exercises.

- **Strength training:** Exercises that work on strength might assist in the recovery of weak muscles and support functions independent of work. Focus on training the major muscle groups of the body, like the leg press and arm curls, and also ensure that you spare some time to strengthen the abdominal muscles.

- **Coordination exercises:** Coordination and motor control might also be ineffective after a stroke. Activities that include playing catch, using the coordination boards, and doing hand-eye coordination exercises stretch that interconnection, enhance motor control, and improve these comprehension skills (Mulhern, 2023).

- **Gait training:** Impairments that lead to an ability to walk often occur after a stroke. Examples of gait training exercises include walking in the correct manner, using an assistive device when necessary, and powering oversteps, step-ups, and step-downs. This practice improves gait mobility so that one can walk comfortably.

- **Cognitive exercises:** Strokes often impact cognitive functions like memory, attention, and time, as well as spacial awareness. Exercise in the cognitive domain using crossword puzzles, memory games, and attention tasks will improve cognitive functioning and mental sharpness.

- **Functional activities practice:** Getting involved in everyday activities where individuals perform routine tasks, such as cooking, dressing, and so forth, will help you regain your independence. The functional skills you learn will largely determine your improved status post-stroke.

- **Flexibility exercises:** Stretching exercises enhance flexibility, laying the groundwork for the muscle tissue to become looser and eventually leading to increased control of the range of motion of the joints. Concentrate on muscular strains related to major muscle groups and muscle tightness to achieve incremental mobility (Mulhern, 2023).

These adaptation training opportunities aid post-stroke patients in rehabilitating themselves from muscle weakness, coordination, balance, mobility problems, cognitive deficit, and returning to a state of self-dependence. It is advisable to seek the advice of your healthcare provider or physiotherapist before embarking on any exercise program to ensure that safety is prioritized. The healthcare team will devise the best routine for each condition.

Creating a Safe Environment

Providing a safe environment for neurovascular recovery is critical for persons after suffering a stroke to reduce the likelihood of mishaps, enable them to be independent, and support their rehabilitation goals. A secure environment can reduce the risk of falling, making it easier to perform everyday activities while facilitating recovery. Here are three to five environmental considerations you should engage in post-stroke:

- **Clear pathways:** Keep personal items like toys and books out of foot traffic areas, and remove rugs and all possible tripping hazards. These could all result in tripping, slipping, or falling, which should be avoided. Keep pathways clear and freely walkable so the individual can move safely post-stroke.

- **Proper lighting:** Proper lighting ensures that everyone, including persons with impaired eyesight or balance post-stroke, is safe during recovery. Provide good illumination and install nightlights or motion-sensor lights, especially on the path to the bathroom (Mulhern, 2023).

- **Grab bars and handrails:** Smooth grab bars and handrails should be installed in critical areas, including bathrooms, stairways, and hallways, to aid the balance and movement of stroke survivors. These devices can help prevent falls and help people move safely through the house.

- **Non-slip surfaces:** Make your bathroom and kitchen safer with non-slip mats or rugs in moist areas. You will increase your chances of avoiding slipping on them. Consider applying anti-slip adhesive strips on stairs and slopes to increase grip or traction, which is necessary to stabilize movement.

- **Accessible furniture and equipment:** Coordinate the placement of furniture and appliances in a manner that will not create obstacles in movement for yourself or someone else who has had a stroke. Ensure that the arrangement enables you to move actively on your own.

This chapter demonstrated the significance of implementing practical and applicable post-stroke strategies that promote cognitive function. These strategies enhance the use of memory to resolve the issue of improving intelligence. This chapter emphasized the practice of reliance on cognitive abilities that promote independence post-stroke. You can achieve all your goals by pursuing individual therapeutic approaches and structured cognitive rehabilitation training programs. Eventually, if you follow these prescribed processes, you can exercise your cognitive potential and improve the quality of your life.

The next chapter will talk about the emotional impact of stroke and ways of promoting mental well-being and resilience. Stroke survivors may suffer from several psychological difficulties, including depression, anxiety, and adjustment difficulties. This chapter underscores the significance of psychological support and self-care as part of the effort to curb emotional problems after a stroke.

Psychological Well-being After a Stroke

Dear self, I know you are doing the best you can. I believe in you. Keep going. Love Me

—Anonymous

We begin this chapter with a heartfelt message that resonates with self-compassion and encouragement. This profound introduction sets the tone for a chapter on the emotional path of stroke recovery and the essential role of psychological well-being. Focusing on self-compassion, resilience, and mental health support, this chapter emphasizes the importance of nurturing emotional well-being post-stroke. Through personal reflections, practical strategies, and insights, it aims to empower individuals to cultivate inner strength, cope with challenges, and lead to a positive outlook on their recovery path.

Dealing with Anxiety and Depression Post-Stroke

Patients may experience depression and anxiety post-stroke due to various factors, including:

- **Biological changes:** Stroke may cause the alteration of brain chemistry and its performance, which might well give rise to the onset of depression and anxiety (American Stroke Association, 2019).

- **Emotional impact:** Motor weakness, sensory problems, and lifestyle changes due to a stroke require a victim to combat depression, hopelessness, and fear (Kirkevold et al., 2018).

- **Social isolation:** Post-stroke, some parts of a person's social life, like communicating and moving around, will become problematic. Those can make the person feel lonely and isolated. Those can result in anxiety and depression (American Stroke Association, 2019).

- **Fear of recurrence:** The anxiety of getting yet another stroke or worse health issues is what stroke survivors have to deal with. Sometimes, this can lead to genuinely troubling anxiety and distress.

Depression

Signs and symptoms/pathognomonic features of depression are:

- Frequently being in a low mood state with a lack of interest and a lost sense of meaning in life.

- Disinclination to take part in activities that used to be of interest.

- Alterations in cravings or weight.

- Sleep problems (in the form of lack of sleep or excessive sleep).

- Fatigue or low energy.

- Distressing phenomena such as lightness of mind or difficulty staying focused and attentive.

- Feelings of regret or shame.

- Death of someone does more harm than just losing a loved one; it can lead to critical thoughts of death or suicide.

Coping with Depression

You can:
- Seek help from a health provider or a mental health care professional.

- Enroll in counseling or psychotherapy

- Conversing with a doctor may help you decide about medication if needed.

- Join the gym, spend time with family and friends, and do activities you enjoy.

- Proper nutrition, sleep, and adequate stress management are also important for good body health.

Anxiety

Anxiety that occurs after a stroke may include worrying quite a lot over the smallest things, being afraid of things that never used to frighten you before and being consumed by fear of what might happen in the future. The physical signs of anxiety are distracted mind, muscle tension, nervousness, and edginess. Like depression after a stroke, anxiety may be reduced using similar techniques, such as seeing a specialist, attending relevant therapy, undertaking relaxation activities, and making sure that one keeps up a healthy lifestyle. Through the appropriate management of depression and anxiety, stroke survivors gain the ability to restore their emotional state and lead better lives when they are grappling with recovery (American Stroke Association, 2019).

Coping with Anxiety

Therapeutic Interventions

- **Cognitive Behavioral Therapy (CBT):** CBT, which is one of the most preferable approaches in therapy, allows people to identify and challenge the negative thoughts and beliefs that lead to anxiety and change. It offers tools to focus on nervous thoughts and take appropriate action (Kirkevold et al., 2018).

- **Mindfulness-Based Stress Reduction (MBSR):** MBSR includes mindfulness meditation and awareness exercises, which, in turn, help train the inner self to live in the present, stress less, and cope with anxiety disorders (American Stroke Association, 2019).

- **Relaxation Techniques:** Methods of introspection, such as deep breathing exercises, progressive muscle relaxation, and guided imagery, are all known for their contributions to relaxation, such as reducing physical tension and eliminating anxiety symptoms.

- **Exposure Therapy:** This psychological technique involves taking clients impacted by anxiety and gradually placing them in a safe and tranquil surrounding, which helps them combat their fears (Kirkevold et al., 2018).

Support Networks

You are encouraged to make good use of the following support networks:

- **Family and friends:** Establishing a solid group of friends and relatives who can help you with emotional reassurance and companionship creates a support network that ushers in a feeling of belonging, reducing emotional isolation.

- **Support groups:** Participation in support groups for stroke survivors and people with anxiety provides a sense of community, and sharing experiences with peers can provide excellent support (American Stroke Association, 2019).

- **Therapeutic relationships:** Through trusting and supportive relationships with either therapist, counselor, or mental health professionals, you can create a safe space for addressing anxiety-related issues.

- **Online communities:** Participating in online forums can offer a platform for people to exchange information, gather advice, and find peer support from those who understand their situation (American Stroke Association, 2019).

An approach that includes therapeutic tools and leaning on networks of support will give individuals with anxiety after a stroke the opportunity to make use of valuable resources, strategies, and contacts. These efforts will help with symptom management and lead to a better lifestyle during the recovery process.

Mental Resilience

Understand how mental resilience, mind-body practices, cognitive behavioral strategies, and setting realistic resilience goals can contribute to psychological well-being after a stroke:

- **Mind-body practices:** Post-stroke, people typically encounter physical and emotional hardship. For example, techniques like mind-body-oriented practices involving meditation, deep breathing, and slow yoga can substantially help recovery. These exercises effectively de-stress, make you feel better, and open up more inner space. The mental and body relaxation that mind-body exercises bring results in better general health and the capacity to cope with adversities for stroke survivors (American Stroke Association, 2019).

- **Cognitive behavioral strategies** (CBT): This is one of the proven cognitive behavioral strategies for stroke patients that is particularly helpful in coping with emotions such as depression, anxiety, and mental adjustments. These approaches are essential because they pinpoint and discredit negative reflections and substitute them with similarly helpful and positive ones. After a stroke, CBT can alleviate challenges experienced in adjusting to the new lifestyle, improve mood, and increase problem-solving abilities (Kirkevold et al., 2018).

- **Setting realistic resilience goals:** To successfully build resilience during rehabilitation, stroke survivors should aim to set reasonable goals they are capable of. This could be accomplished by identifying their problems, e.g., physical limitations, cognitive impairments, emotional difficulty, etc. Lastly, creating practical tools to solve those problems is something you should be doing. By setting some doable targets, stroke survivors can sit with self-belief, gradually feeling in charge of their affairs and developing better mental health.

- **Overall improvement in mental resilience:** When put together, the efforts mentioned above can help immensely in building the resilience of stroke survivors. While mind-body practices supply control techniques for stress and encourage relaxation, cognitive behavioral strategy is employed to deal with negative feelings and distorted beliefs. By establishing actionable practices for improving resilience, stroke survivors are motivated to initiate the recovery process and the alterations in lifestyle they have to live with when they suffer from a stroke. The aggregate effect of these interventions enables a higher level of resilience, good health, and a better quality of life.

Understanding Personality Changes

Neurological reorganization after a stroke often causes changes in personality such as altered mood, behavior, and interpersonal interactions. Some would be more seemingly irritable, impulsive, or apathetic. Some of them can cause mood changes, depression, and anxiety. The shift in personality could also differ drastically depending on the type of stroke.

Signs to Look Out For

The most evident symptoms of personality changes that appear after stroke include uneven mood swings, emotional changes that lead to increased agitation, lack of empathy, sudden impulsive actions, and problems socializing with others. These will likely be psychological and neurological signs, some of which could be hidden. Thus, everybody, especially caretakers and family, should be aware of these subtle signs as they may indicate underlying psychological or neurological changes.

Communication Strategies

You have to employ effective strategic communication to better interact with post-stroke individuals whose personality changes have negatively impacted them. These may include:

- **Patience and understanding:** Display patience and empathy; be aware that the individual's behavior is beyond their control. You need to exercise patience and listen carefully when communicating with patients recovering from stroke.

- **Clear and simple language:** By using brief and comprehensible sentence construction, you can further increase understanding and clarity.

- **Active listening:** Listen to the individual to portray empathy and validate their feelings and experiences.

During stroke recovery, consider the nature of personality changes, be careful to notice possible signs, and use efficient communication methods to help the sick person and the caregiver work together and improve their relationship.

Managing Stress

Stress management should remain the priority during stroke recovery. Here's how to understand stress during recovery, de-stress techniques, and incorporating mindfulness into daily life:

- **Understanding stress during recovery:** Handling a stroke effectively is physically and psychologically draining. Therefore, the level of stress can become very high. Stroke patients may have lost physical abilities, are taking new medications, and are dealing with emotional effects. Acknowledging and understanding these burdening factors enables families or individuals to take measures to manage their stress levels.

- **De-stressing techniques:** To manage stress during stroke recovery, muscle relaxation techniques consist of sequentially tensing and relaxing different muscle groups so that tension is released and people de-stress and relax (Kirkevold et al., 2018). Specific breathing techniques involve deep breathing, which can help a patient become relaxed and, as a result, reduce stress levels.

- **Incorporating mindfulness into daily life:** The practice of mindfulness requires that individuals focus their attention on the present without evaluating their emotional state. This truth can be particularly beneficial as a simple management technique when managing stress during stroke recovery.

When learning to cope with stress during the recovery process, techniques to de-stress can be implemented, and mindfulness can be incorporated into everyday life. Such practices will enable individuals to turn the tide and help them reduce their stress levels while improving the quality of their recovery program (American Stroke Association, 2019).

This chapter aimed to scrutinize the psychosocial impact of psychological health post-stroke, thus examining the emotional, cognitive, and social aspects that transpire in an individual. You learned about how a variety of mental health issues are brought on by stroke, such as depression, anxiety, and post-stroke adjustment disorders. Confronting such psychological issues involves developing different strategies for coping as well as intervention approaches to facilitate recovery and enhance long-term psychological strengthening.

Chapter 8 shifts to overall health strategies and community programs for stroke patients to improve their quality of life. This chapter encourages them to make lifestyle changes and includes issues such as healthy diet, exercise, stress management, social interaction for maximum power, and mental health.

Lifestyle Modifications for Optimal Health

If you know you can alter your lifestyle, diet, and avoid heart disease as well as other things, you should do it.

–Laila Ali

Heart disease and stroke are largely lifestyle diseases. You can change your disease pathway by changing your lifestyle and adopting healthier habits. Chapter 8 details the life-altering number of lifestyle adjustments that encourage post-rehabilitation recovery and general health. Inspired by Laila Ali's quote, this chapter underscores the profound impact of proactive changes in diet, exercise, and daily habits on mitigating risks associated with heart disease and other health concerns. It advocates for a holistic approach to health, emphasizing the integration of physical activity, nutrition, stress management, and social engagement into daily routines. By empowering individuals with practical strategies and personalized plans, Chapter 8 aims to facilitate a smooth transition from rehabilitation to a vibrant, fulfilling life, where proactive lifestyle modifications serve as pillars of long-term health and vitality.

Adopting a Heart-Healthy Diet

This is a book about stroke recovery. Why are we discussing heart health? A heart-healthy diet is really just a diet that is healthy for your blood vessels, which traverse your entire body. Your arteries don't know the organs to which they are supplying blood. A heart-healthy diet is also a brain-healthy diet. Adopting a heart-healthy diet during rehabilitation plays a pivotal role in promoting recovery and preventing future health issues, especially considering the potential impact of diet on stroke occurrence. By being mindful and conscious of what you eat, you can address dietary factors that might have contributed to the stroke and positively change your overall health (Bailey, 2018).

Reassessing Your Perception of Food

Reasons to reevaluate your perception of food include:

- **Nutritional impact:** Recognizing that food is fuel for your body enables you to understand the importance of consuming nutrient-dense foods to support recovery and overall health.

- **Long-term health:** Embracing a balanced diet increases long-term health benefits, reducing the risk of future strokes and other cardiovascular diseases.

- **Mental well-being:** Understanding the connection between diet and mental health will enable you to appreciate how wholesome foods can positively impact mood and cognitive function.

Healthy relationships with food involve prioritizing whole, unprocessed foods rich in nutrients while being mindful of portion sizes. In contrast, unhealthy relationships with food often involve reliance on fast food or convenience foods, which may provide short-term satisfaction but lack essential nutrients and contribute to poor health outcomes.

Whole Foods

Whole foods refer to natural, unprocessed foods that are minimally refined or altered from their original state. These foods are typically nutrient-dense and provide essential vitamins, minerals, fiber, and other beneficial nutrients in their natural form. Whole foods include fruits, vegetables, whole grains, nuts, seeds, legumes, lean proteins, and unprocessed meats. Unlike processed foods, which often contain additives, preservatives, and artificial ingredients, whole foods retain their nutritional integrity and offer numerous health benefits. Integrating a variety of whole foods into one's diet can support overall health, aid in weight management, and reduce the risk of chronic diseases such as heart disease, diabetes, and stroke (Bailey, 2018).

Good and Bad Fats

Good fats, also known as unsaturated fats, are beneficial for heart health and can help lower cholesterol levels when consumed in moderation. They include monounsaturated fats and polyunsaturated fats. These fats are typically liquid at room temperature and are found in nuts, seeds, avocados, and fatty fish (Bailey, 2018).

Bad fats, also known as saturated and trans fats, can raise cholesterol levels and increase the risk of heart disease when consumed in excess.

Saturated fats are mainly found in animal products such as butter, cheese, fatty meats, and plant-based oils like coconut and palm oil. Trans fats are primarily found in processed foods like fried foods, baked goods, and margarine.

Cholesterol plays a role in the body's cell structure and hormone production. But, high levels of LDL (low-density lipoprotein) cholesterol, often referred to as "bad" cholesterol, can contribute to the buildup of plaque in the arteries, increasing the risk of heart disease and strokes. Good fats, such as polyunsaturated and monounsaturated fats, can help lower LDL cholesterol levels, while bad fats, such as saturated and trans fats, can raise LDL cholesterol levels.

Three good fats and how to integrate them into daily life are:

- **Avocado:** Add sliced avocado to salads, sandwiches, or smoothies for a creamy texture and healthy fats.

- **Nuts (e.g., almonds, walnuts, pistachios):** Snack on a handful of mixed nuts, sprinkle them over yogurt or oatmeal, or incorporate them into a homemade trail mix.

- **Fatty fish (e.g., salmon, mackerel, sardines):** Grill or bake fish fillets for a nutritious main dish, or add canned salmon or tuna to salads, wraps, or pasta dishes.

Three bad fats and alternatives to them are:

- **Butter:** Replace butter with healthier alternatives like olive oil, avocado oil, or nut-based spreads like almond butter or cashew butter.

- **Processed meats (e.g., bacon, sausage, hot dogs):** Opt for lean cuts of meat, like skinless poultry, fish, or plant-based protein sources like tofu or legumes.

- **Full-fat dairy products (e.g., whole milk, cheese, cream):** Choose low-fat or fat-free dairy options like skim milk, reduced-fat cheese, or Greek yogurt.

Exercise Plan

Cardio Exercises to Promote a Healthy Heart

Do the following routines:

- **Brisk walking:** Aim for at least 30 minutes of brisk walking most days of the week.

- **Cycling:** Ride a bike outdoors or use a stationary bike for 30-60 minutes, 3-5 times per week.

- **Swimming:** Swim laps in a pool or engage in water aerobics for 30-45 minutes, 3-4 times per week.

- **Jumping rope:** Perform 10-15 minutes of jumping rope intervals 3-4 times per week.

- **Dancing:** Take dance classes or dance to your favorite music for 30-45 minutes, 2-3 times per week (Saunders et al., 2021).

Strength Training Exercises to Promote a Healthy Heart

Engage in the upcoming workouts:

- **Bodyweight squats:** Perform 2-3 sets of 10-15 repetitions each, 2-3 times per week.

- **Push-ups:** Do 2-3 sets of 8-12 repetitions each, 2-3 times per week. You can start with wall push-ups, progress to prone push-ups on your knees, and finally on your toes.

- **Dumbbell or kettlebell lunges:** Complete 2-3 sets of 10-12 repetitions per leg, 2-3 times per week.

- **Resistance band rows:** Perform 2-3 sets of 10-15 repetitions each, 2-3 times per week.

- **Planks:** Hold a plank position for 30-60 seconds, 2-3 times per week.

- **Dumbbell or kettlebell deadlifts:** Do 2-3 sets of 8-12 repetitions each, 2-3 times per week.

- **Medicine ball slams:** Perform 2-3 sets of 10-15 repetitions each, 2-3 times per week (Saunders et al., 2021).

Sleep

The average person should aim for 7-9 hours of sleep per night for optimal health and well-being.

Why Does Sleep Matter?

Sleep is crucial during post-stroke recovery and vital in facilitating physical and cognitive healing processes. Adequate sleep promotes neuroplasticity, the brain's ability to rewire and repair itself, which is essential for lost function and learning new skills after a stroke. Furthermore, sleep is crucial for mood regulation, memory consolidation, and immune function, all of which are integral to recovery. Post-stroke sleep disturbances such as insomnia, sleep apnea, or disrupted sleep patterns are to be expected due to physical discomfort, psychological distress, or changes in brain function (Bailey, 2018).

Creating a Sleep Routine

A sleep routine is a set of activities performed before bedtime to promote restful and uninterrupted sleep.

What Makes a Good Sleep Routine?

The upcoming techniques enable a sufficient bedtime routine:

- **Consistent bedtime:** Going to bed and waking up at the same time every day helps regulate the body's internal clock, promoting better sleep quality and duration.

- **Relaxation techniques:** Engaging in relaxation practices such as deep breathing, meditation, or gentle stretching before bed can help calm the mind and body, making it easier to fall asleep.

- **Limiting screen time:** Avoiding electronic devices such as smartphones, tablets, and computers at least an hour before bedtime helps reduce exposure to blue light, which can disrupt the body's natural sleep-wake cycle.

- **Creating a comfortable environment:** Ensure the bedroom is dark, quiet, and at a comfortable temperature to promote relaxation and minimize disturbances during sleep.

- **Avoiding stimulants:** Limiting caffeine and alcohol consumption, especially before bedtime, can prevent sleep disturbances and promote deeper, more restorative sleep. The caffeine in one cup of coffee will stay in your system for 6 hours. Count backwards from the time that you'd like to go to sleep and don't drink any caffeinated beverages after that time.

- **Establishing a bedtime routine:** Before bed, engage in calming activities such as reading, taking a warm bath, or listening to soothing music to signal to the body that it's time to wind down and prepare for sleep.

- **Regular exercise:** Incorporating regular physical activity into your daily routine can promote better sleep quality and help alleviate symptoms of insomnia or sleep disturbances. However, avoid vigorous exercise close to bedtime, as it may interfere with sleep.

Sleep Disorders

- **Sleep apnea:** A condition characterized by pauses in breathing during sleep, often accompanied by loud snoring and daytime sleepiness. Sleep apnea causes sudden drops in oxygen levels, straining the cardiovascular system. You may not realize that you have sleep apnea as you won't fully awaken during these episodes.

- **Restless Legs Syndrome (RLS):** Uncomfortable sensations in the legs, typically occurring at night and causing an irresistible urge to move the legs.

- **Narcolepsy:** A neurological disorder characterized by excessive daytime sleepiness and sudden episodes of falling asleep during the day.

- **REM Sleep Behavior Disorder (RBD):** Acting out vivid and often violent dreams during REM sleep, potentially causing injury to oneself or a bed partner.

- **Insomnia:** Difficulty falling or staying asleep, leading to insufficient rest and daytime fatigue. Insomnia can be exacerbated by depression and anxiety.

Post-Stroke vs. Pre-Stroke Sleep Disorders

Sleep disorders can occur both pre-stroke and post-stroke. However, strokes can exacerbate or contribute to the development of sleep disorders due to factors such as changes in brain function, physical limitations, or psychological distress resulting from the stroke. For example, strokes can lead to disruptions in the brain's sleep-wake cycle, causing insomnia or sleep apnea. Physical impairments or discomfort post-stroke may exacerbate restless legs syndrome.

Addressing Sleep Disorders

Treatment for sleep disorders often involves a combination of lifestyle modifications, behavioral therapy, and medical interventions. Depending on the specific sleep disorder, treatment options may include:

- Lifestyle changes, such as maintaining a regular sleep schedule, practicing relaxation techniques, and avoiding caffeine and alcohol before bedtime.

- Continuous positive airway pressure (CPAP) therapy for sleep apnea (Bailey, 2018).

- Medications such as sedatives, antidepressants, or medications to manage symptoms of restless legs syndrome. Sedative sleep aids can be addictive, so use them as a last resort.

- Cognitive-behavioral therapy (CBT) for insomnia focuses on changing negative thoughts and behaviors related to sleep.

Social Connections - Why They Matter

Social connections are essential for overall well-being and quality of life, especially during post-stroke recovery. Maintaining social connections can:

- **Provide emotional support:** Social relationships offer emotional support, encouragement, and companionship, which are vital in coping with the challenges of a stroke and promoting mental health (Hoffman, 2017).

- **Facilitate rehabilitation:** Engaging in social activities and interactions can enhance motivation, confidence, and participation in rehabilitation efforts, leading to better outcomes in physical and cognitive recovery.

- **Combat feelings of isolation:** Social connections help combat feelings of loneliness and isolation commonly experienced after a stroke, promoting a sense of belonging and connectedness within one's community.

- **Promote mental health:** Positive social interactions and relationships contribute to improved mood, self-esteem, and overall psychological well-being, reducing the risk of depression and anxiety post-stroke.

- **Encourage healthy behaviors:** Social support networks can encourage healthy lifestyle behaviors, such as exercise, dietary changes, and medication adherence, which are crucial for stroke prevention and management.

Nurturing social connections and maintaining meaningful relationships is essential for promoting emotional well-being, facilitating recovery, and enhancing stroke survivors' overall quality of life.

Importance of Reconnecting with Friends and Family

You need to understand the importance of reconnecting with family and friends by reviewing the information below.

- **Emotional support:** Friends and family provide a valuable support network that offers empathy, encouragement, and understanding during challenging times, such as post-stroke recovery (Hoffman, 2017).

- **Reduced isolation:** Humans are social creatures. Social connections help combat loneliness and isolation, promoting a sense of belonging and connectedness within one's community.

- **Improved mental health:** Reconnecting with loved ones can boost one's mood, reduce stress, and alleviate symptoms of depression and anxiety, contributing to better overall mental health and well-being (Hoffman, 2017).

- **Enhanced quality of life:** Meaningful relationships with friends and family enrich life experiences, bring joy and fulfillment, and provide a sense of purpose and meaning (Saunders et al., 2021).

- **Facilitated recovery:** Social support networks can enhance motivation, adherence to treatment plans, and engagement in rehabilitation efforts, leading to better outcomes in physical and cognitive recovery.

Activities that Promote Connectedness

The following activities encourage connectedness:

- **Social gatherings:** To foster camaraderie and bonding, organize small get-togethers with friends and family, such as potluck dinners, game nights, or movie marathons (Saunders et al., 2021).

- **Community events:** Attend local community events, festivals, or cultural celebrations with friends or family to engage with others and connect with the broader community.

- **Group exercise classes:** Join group exercise classes or recreational sports leagues to stay active while socializing and building connections with like-minded individuals.

- **Volunteer work:** Participate in volunteer activities or community service projects with friends or family members to positively impact the community while bonding over shared experiences.

- **Family dinners or outings:** Plan regular family dinners or outings, such as picnics, hikes, or day trips, to strengthen family bonds, create lasting memories, and enjoy quality time together.

In conclusion, Chapter 8 underscores the life-altering potential of lifestyle modifications in promoting optimal health and well-being post-stroke. By embracing healthy habits encompassing diet, exercise, stress management, and social engagement, individuals can enhance their physical, cognitive, and emotional resilience, creating a vibrant and fulfilling life after rehabilitation. Recognizing the interconnections of lifestyle factors in stroke recovery, personalized strategies, and proactive approaches are emphasized to empower individuals toward long-term health sustenance.

Moving on to Chapter 9, the focus shifts towards proactive measures and interventions to reduce the risk of recurrent strokes. This chapter explores strategies for stroke prevention through lifestyle modifications, medical management, and targeted interventions tailored to fulfill individual needs and risk factors.

PREVENTION OF FUTURE STROKES

We often spend a lot of our time doing things that are not particularly wanted, next time just droop the great oil of your heart for just a few moments.

–Anonymous

This chapter stresses that learning from hardships minimizes the risk of having another stroke. Influenced by the opening quote above, it discloses the significance of vascular disease's impact on an individual and the best measures to prevent recurrent strokes.

Each of these actions, such as taking medication as prescribed, dietary changes, exercise routines, stress management techniques, and regular medical check-ups, are essential steps towards averting the occurrence of strokes later on in life. One can make this possible by committing one's heart and soul to achieving optimal health and being confident in one's ability to attain a healthier, happier life with fewer chances of having recurrent strokes (CDC, 2023).

Identifying and Managing Risks

Many stroke cases are due to underlying causes, like:

- **High blood pressure (Hypertension):** High blood pressure is one of the most prevalent risk factors for stroke. Over time it damages the endothelium, the inner lining of blood vessels, leading to clot formation or vessel hemorrhage.

- **Atrial fibrillation (AFib):** Irregular heart rhythm can lead to clot formation inside the heart. If the clot is ejected from the heart, it can strike the brain, causing an embolic stroke.

- **High cholesterol:** An abundance of LDL cholesterol in the system can result in the development of plaque formation, which can lead to an increased risk of stroke due to plaque in the arteries (CDC, 2023).

- **Diabetes:** If uncontrolled, high blood sugars put you at risk of having damaged cardiovascular and nervous systems, eventually leading to a devastating stroke and/or a heart attack.

- **Smoking:** Smoking is not good for the health of blood vessels and other parts of the cardiovascular system, as it damages the arteries and veins, increases blood pressure, and causes the formation of blood clots.

Lifestyle Modifications

It is crucial to make lifestyle changes to prevent future strokes. Below are some fundamental alterations you can implement.

Nutrition

The following dietary stipulations are critical for stroke survivors:

- **Eat for healthy blood vessels:** Adhering to a diet rich in fruits, vegetables, whole grains, lean proteins, and healthy fats (such as those found in fish, nuts, and olive oil) will protect your endothelium, lower blood pressure, and decrease the risk of future strokes (CDC, 2023).

- **Reducing sodium intake:** Eating only natural, unprocessed foods, and avoiding salty snacks is a great way to build good blood pressure and prevent the risk of a stroke.

- **Limiting saturated and trans fats:** Eliminating consumption of foods, namely fried foods, pastries, and processed meats, which have highly saturated and trans fats, can help bring cholesterol levels down and prevent atherosclerosis and stroke (CDC, 2023).

Physical Activity

Implement the following physical workouts:

- **Regular exercise:** To quickly recover and avoid future strokes, moderate-intensity aerobic exercise, such as brisk walking, cycling, and swimming, for at least 150 minutes per week, helps to reduce blood pressure, improve cholesterol levels, and reduce the probability of a stroke.

- **Strength training:** Strength training exercises like lifting weights or using resistance bands can be immensely helpful for better cardiovascular health and reducing the risk of stroke. Also, integrating them into your exercise program for at least two days a week would be highly beneficial (CDC, 2023).

- **Maintaining a healthy weight**: Another method to help reduce the risk of stroke and heart disease is to persist in daily physical activities and maintain a well-balanced diet, free of processed foods.

Recognizing and controlling common stroke risk factors (such as hypertension and diabetes) and applying healthy lifestyle modification can help you slash the odds of having a stroke and considerably improve your cardiovascular health.

Celebrating Milestones and Gains

Acknowledging milestones and gains in recovery is essential for stroke survivors; the following information is vital for you.

Recovery from Stroke

- **Regaining motor function:** Attaining the ability to walk on your own two feet, gaining lost control of hand movements, or improving your balance and coordination are worthwhile achievements of stroke recovery (CDC, 2023).

- **Cognitive improvements:** Landmarks like improved memory, attention, and problem-solving skills show the progress you are making in the rehabilitation process after suffering a stroke.

- **Independence in activities of daily living (ADLs):** Milestones, such as the ability to dress yourself, cook, and manage your personal hygiene, are telltale signs of autonomy and functional recovery after stroke (CDC, 2023).

Tracking Progress and Goals

Highlighting SMART (Specific, Measurable, Achievable, Relevant, Time-bound) goals in stroke recovery is essential for several reasons:

- **Clarity:** SMART goals help people effectively work on specific areas of improvement during the recovery process while seeking to attain their goals with clarity and direction.

- **Measurability:** Measurable targets will help the individual have a clear plan and be able to check on their performances during the path to recovery and success.

- **Motivation:** The ability to develop attainable goals relevant to the rehabilitation process can provide motivation and a feeling of achievement. These are the essential elements in recovery, playing the role of an engine that drives and powers the recovery process further.

- **Accountability:** Establishing deadlines and considering time frames gives you the feeling of responsibility needed to stay on the prearranged healing path within your recovery plan.

Struggles

Prepare for the path to recovery by fighting against the struggles mentioned below:

- **Old habits die hard:** It can be difficult to break old habits. When there is a lot of anxiety and stress, many people are tempted to return to their old lifestyles. Think of ways to make the new habits the path of least resistance.

- **Lack of support:** A lack of family, friends, and medical providers can disorient and isolate you, leading to failure to establish permanent, healthy habits and maintain focus.

- **Plateaus and setbacks:** Although common, plateaus or failures in the recovery process can be demotivating and give way to feelings of irritation or incompetence.

Making Change Easier

The following techniques are essential for making a smooth change:

- **Create a supportive environment:** Avoid toxic people hindering your progress towards a healthy lifestyle. Instead, live among loving friends who inspire you to follow a healthy pattern.

- **Set realistic expectations:** Be aware that failures are typical during the recovery period, and don't get attached to the idea of living life without failures. Failures are a part of life! Use them as opportunities of learning.

Medications

During recovery from a stroke, several types of medications may be prescribed to address various aspects of the condition and prevent future complications:

- **Blood thinners (anticoagulants):** Warfarin is one medication used to prevent blood clots and reduce the possibility of a stroke. Other drugs, such as dabigatran or rivaroxaban, might also be prescribed, especially for patients with atrial fibrillation or a history of clot-related strokes.

- **Antiplatelet agents:** Medicines like aspirin, clopidogrel, or dipyridamole may be included in the treatment plan to manage arterial plaques that could cause ischemic strokes by inhibiting platelet aggregation.

- **Blood pressure medications:** Antihypertensive drugs, including ACE inhibitors, beta-blockers, calcium channel blockers, or diuretics, could be administered to patients to treat high blood pressure, a condition that increases the probability of stroke.

- **Medications for symptom management:** Depending on whether the patient has such problems, medications like antidepressants, muscle relaxants, and medications to reduce spasticity or treat neuropathy can be part of the prescription regimen and improve quality of life during recovery.

Physicals

Medical examinations, which are common to health matters, examine the patient and determine the functionality of all aspects of health, their physical strength, and physical abilities. These often entail obtaining the patient's blood pressure, waistline circumference, and weight and taking blood samples to measure lipid and blood sugar levels in the blood.

Physical examination is the foundation of health assessment because it helps healthcare professionals understand current health status and develop focused treatment plans. Healthcare providers will monitor progress during regular health checks, highlighting areas that have improved, detecting those that need improvement, and allowing for fine-tuning of treatment protocols to maximize recovery and rehabilitation goals. Further, by screening for any hidden health concerns that may affect recovery, professionals can detect and prevent issues that might arise later.

Continuing Your Recovery

Staying in the strategically tailored treatment plan created by your caregivers entails commitment, even once the initial set of interventions has finished. This is conventionally done by engaging in workout regimens, attending therapy sessions, taking medications as prescribed, and implementing necessary lifestyle changes. Consistency and dedication are essential in avoiding disruptions and maintaining constant progress within the system. Frequent consultations and information sharing with healthcare providers are necessary to ensure that routines are appropriate and change accordingly as the patient improves.

In this chapter, you learned that stroke prevention entirely depends on proactive measures that need to be taken. Through lifestyle changes, managing risk factors such as hypertension, diabetes, and cholesterol, and adherence to prescriptions, you can reduce the chances of a new stroke occurring in your future. Education and awareness are pivotal, as they will be a source of information that help turn the tide and help people stay in control of their health, thus preventing all stroke-related complications. Through resolve and dedication to preventative measures, you may attain a safer health situation with a much lower risk of stroke while achieving better health. Chapter 10 aims to guide stroke survivors through life after a stroke and identify the path towards a healthy life.

Living a Fulfilling Life Post-Stroke

You have only one trustworthy gateway, so take good care of its health. It is no demand to consider your favorite commodity valuable. Instead, give time to your most essential possession, which is your health.

–Unknown

The goal is to find independence after a stroke. Healthcare professionals call it returning to your prior state of health. As we've mentioned before, heart disease and strokes are caused by poor lifestyle. In reality, the true goal is to improve upon your prior state of health.

When facing challenges, you must stand on your own two feet and be autonomous. You also have to learn to interact with others and understand how much support you need from them. While seeking the support of those around you, it's important to know just how much of it you need.

To understand how much help you need, you must learn to communicate effectively; this chapter will guide you on how to achieve this. Finally, this chapter will teach you the tricks of getting ready to return to work and how others can prepare a good work environment that meets your needs as a stroke survivor.

Reclaiming Independence

Reclaiming independence involves:

- **Rehabilitation therapies:** Physical, occupational, and speech therapy are used to improve motor skills, cognitive function, and communication abilities (Dongen et al., 2021).

- **Assistive devices:** A stroke survivor can reclaim independence by using mobility aids, communication tools, or adaptive equipment to increase self-sufficiency in daily life.

- **Home modifications:** Medical equipment designed to adjust to each person's unique living environment can help overcome physical challenges while staying safe and accessible (Dongen et al., 2021).

- **Personalized goals:** Create attainable goals and work on them to improve self-control and confidence within a stroke survivor.

- **Social support:** Develop connections with family members, friends, and healthcare professionals who can share ideas and offer support throughout the recovery process and beyond.

Gaining independence is crucial to recovery, as it boosts your feelings of discipline, respect, and purpose. It enables you to actively participate in daily chores, increase self-sufficiency, and live a complete life. A study conducted in elderly homes showed residents with pets were happier and socialized more with their furry friends, enabling them to be independent. Becoming independent again can lead to increased self-confidence, motivation, and resilience, allowing such people to live better lives post-stroke, resulting in long-term recovery (Dongen et al., 2021).

How Others Can Support

Those around you can support your efforts to regain independence in the following ways:

- **Encouragement and motivation:** Encouraging inspirational words, compliments, and motivation will help boost your confidence when necessary.

- **Assistance with daily tasks:** Providing simple daily assistance such as preparing food, household chores, transportation, or personal care will be a great relief and promote recovery (Dongen et al., 2021).

- **Participation in therapy sessions:** A critical component of any rehabilitation process is ensuring that the loved ones of those dealing with stroke recovery are actively involved. Attending therapy sessions with a family member, participating in exercises or practice activities, and offering feedback can significantly enhance the effectiveness of rehabilitation efforts.

- **Creating a supportive environment:** Ensuring changes to the living space to better address mobility, safety, and comfort and reducing hindrance factors to enhance independence are key to creating fast recovery and determining autonomy.

- **Education and advocacy:** Knowledge of stroke recovery

processes, realizing how everyone can understand each other's needs and limitations, and providing the necessary facilities and support services empower the individual and their support network (Dongen et al., 2021).

How to Encourage Others to Support You

To get your support system to support you, you can:

- **Communicate openly**: Share what you need, want, and desire within your network so that each individual will understand your issues while you jointly take charge of the recovery process.

- **Provide education and resources:** Get them excited to commit their support to you by transmitting information about stroke recovery, treatment options, and available support services to the group so that you can get their involvement and help.

- **Foster mutual understanding:** Encourage dialogue, listen actively, and have the compassion that will help others understand your plight and give you appropriate assistance (Dongen et al., 2021).

These relationships and support systems are special because they provide various forms of assistance, understanding, and validation essential for navigating the complexities of recovery and rehabilitation. They offer a sense of belonging, empathy, and encouragement, significantly enhancing resilience and encouraging positive outcomes. They also create opportunities for personal growth, learning, and meaningful connections, contributing to long-term wellness.

How to Communicate Your Needs and Wants

Here are six communication techniques, along with example statements, to help communicate your needs and wants effectively:

- **Be Assertive:** "I need some quiet time to rest and recharge. Could you please keep the noise level down?"

- **Use "I" Statements:** "I feel overwhelmed with my current workload. I need help prioritizing tasks to manage them effectively."

- **Be Specific:** "I want to attend therapy sessions twice a week to address my anxiety symptoms."

- **Active Listening**: "I understand that you're busy, but I really need someone to talk to right now. Could you spare a few minutes to listen?"

- **Express Gratitude:** "Thank you for your support so far. I really appreciate it."

- **Create Boundaries:** "At this point, I am unable to do that. Moving forward, I need you to respect my boundaries regarding my recovery process."

These communication techniques can help individuals effectively express their needs and wants, fostering understanding and collaboration within their support systems.

Resources and Support to Consider

Here are seven resources and support systems that can aid in recovery and rehabilitation:

- **Professional healthcare services:** Accessing healthcare professionals such as doctors, therapists, counselors, and rehabilitation specialists can provide tailored treatment plans, medical support, and therapeutic interventions to address specific needs.

- **Support groups:** Joining support groups for individuals experiencing similar challenges can offer empathy, shared experiences, and practical advice. Whether in-person or online, support groups provide a sense of community and reduce feelings of isolation.

- **Community centers and nonprofit organizations:** Community centers and nonprofit organizations often offer a variety of resources and programs, including wellness workshops, fitness classes, educational seminars, and support services tailored to individuals undergoing rehabilitation.

- **Rehabilitation facilities:** Rehabilitation facilities provide comprehensive programs and therapies for individuals recovering from neurological and physical injuries, surgeries, or medical illnesses. These facilities offer structured support, medical supervision, and specialized treatments to promote physical and mental healing (CDC, 2023).

- **Peer mentoring programs:** Engaging with peer mentoring programs connects individuals with mentors who have successfully navigated similar recovery journeys. Peer mentors offer guidance, encouragement, and practical strategies based on their experiences, inspiring hope and fostering resilience.

- **Online resources and mobile apps:** Numerous online resources and mobile apps are designed to support recovery and rehabilitation. These platforms offer educational materials, self-help tools, tracking features, and virtual support networks accessible anytime, anywhere (CDC, 2023).

- **Family and social support networks:** Leveraging the support of family members, friends, and social networks can provide emotional, financial, and practical assistance throughout the recovery process. These relationships offer unconditional love, encouragement, and companionship, which is essential for encouraging resilience and well-being.

Preparing for the Return to Work

- **Review work responsibilities:** Familiarize yourself with job duties, projects, and any changes during your absence.

- **Communicate with your employer:** Discuss return-to-work arrangements, including schedules, accommodations, and any concerns you may have.

- **Organize personal affairs:** Arrange childcare, transportation, and other logistical considerations to ensure a smooth transition (CDC, 2023).

- **Update skills:** Refresh your knowledge and skills related to your role or industry to enhance productivity and effectiveness.

- **Set realistic expectations:** Acknowledge that returning to work may bring challenges and setbacks, and be prepared to adapt gradually.

Considerations When Returning to Work

- **Health and safety:** Assess workplace safety protocols, if applicable, to ensure a safe environment upon returning to work.

- **Emotional well-being:** Recognize and address any emotional or mental health concerns related to returning to work and seeking support.

- **Work-life balance:** Consider adjustments to maintain a healthy work-life balance, prioritizing self-care and boundaries to prevent burnout.

Transition Planning Post-stroke

Transition planning post-stroke involves preparing and coordinating the steps necessary for a smooth and successful transition from acute care settings to rehabilitation and eventually going home or another safe environment for a stroke survivor. This process focuses on assessing the individual's needs, setting goals for recovery, identifying resources and support systems, and developing strategies to facilitate adjustment to life after stroke (CDC, 2023).

Having a transition plan post-stroke helps in several ways:

- **Facilitates continuity of care:** Transition planning ensures a coordinated and seamless transition between different phases of care, such as acute hospital care, rehabilitation, and home care. This helps maintain continuity of medical treatment, therapy, and support services.

- **Addresses individual needs:** The transition plan is tailored to the specific needs and goals of the stroke survivor, taking into account factors such as physical impairments, cognitive deficits, communication difficulties, and emotional challenges (CDC, 2023).

- **Promotes independence and functional recovery:** A well-developed transition plan includes strategies to encourage independence and functional recovery post-stroke. This may involve setting rehabilitation goals, identifying assistive devices or technologies, and providing training for activities of daily living.

- **Supports caregivers and family members:** Transition planning also considers the needs of caregivers and family members who may be involved in the stroke survivor's care. It provides them with information, resources, and support to assist in the transition process and cope with the challenges of caregiving (CDC, 2023).

- **Prevents hospital readmissions:** A comprehensive transition plan aims to reduce the risk of hospital readmissions by addressing factors such as medication management, follow-up care, and lifestyle modifications to prevent complications post-stroke.

A transition plan post-stroke is essential for ensuring continuity of care, addressing individual needs, promoting independence and functional recovery, supporting caregivers, and preventing complications and readmissions. Without a transition plan, stroke survivors and their families may face challenges in accessing appropriate care and resources, leading to poorer outcomes and increased burden on both the individual and their caregivers.

New Norms or Realities Post-Stroke

- **Physical impairments:** Individuals may experience changes in mobility, strength, coordination, and sensation due to stroke-related damage to the brain and nervous system (CDC, 2023).

- **Cognitive challenges:** Stroke survivors may encounter difficulties with memory, attention, problem-solving, and information processing, which can impact various aspects of daily functionality.

- **Emotional changes:** Mood swings, depression, anxiety, and emotional lability are common post-stroke, affecting emotional well-being and interpersonal relationships.

- **Life adjustments:** Stroke survivors may need to adapt to new roles, routines, and lifestyle modifications to accommodate physical and cognitive limitations to optimize recovery. Caregivers will also need to adapt to new roles and responsibilities.

Redefining Your New Reality

Reflecting on your pre-stroke life and life during stroke and then finding the best way to factor in lifestyle modifications can help stroke survivors and their caregivers redefine their new reality. The following are some key techniques that you can adopt:

- **Physical rehabilitation:** Revisit strategies and exercises recommended by healthcare professionals to promote physical recovery and mobility post-stroke. Incorporate adaptive techniques and assistive devices to optimize independence and function (CDC, 2023).

- **Cognitive rehabilitation:** Review cognitive exercises, memory aids, and compensatory strategies introduced during cognitive rehabilitation sessions—practice techniques to enhance memory, attention, problem-solving, and communication skills in daily life.

- **Emotional well-being:** Prioritize self-care and emotional support by connecting with friends, family, support groups, and mental health professionals: practice stress management techniques, mindfulness, and relaxation exercises to cope with emotional challenges post-stroke.

- **Lifestyle modifications:** Implement lifestyle modifications discussed in previous chapters, such as dietary changes, medication management, exercise routines, and sleep hygiene practices, to support overall health and well-being post-stroke.

By redefining their new reality and embracing adjustments, stroke survivors and their caregivers can navigate the challenges of life post-stroke with resilience, hope, and determination.

Embracing adjustments and redefining one's new reality is essential for stroke survivors to lead fulfilling lives. By adapting to physical, cognitive, and emotional changes, individuals can navigate challenges with resilience and optimism, engaging in rehabilitation efforts and incorporating lifestyle modifications to optimize recovery outcomes.

The last chapter discusses emerging trends, technologies, and research in stroke rehabilitation, offering insights into innovative approaches and promising advancements shaping the future of stroke care. From cutting-edge therapies to holistic support systems, this chapter explores the evolving landscape of stroke recovery, inspiring hope, and possibilities for enhanced quality of life post-stroke.

The Future of Stroke Recovery

Technology is anything that wasn't around when you were born.
—Alan Kay

This part of the book goes into the exciting world of improvements in technology and research, defining the subject of stroke recovery. As technology evolves, so does the capacity for creative interventions and therapies to improve recovery results post-stroke. From robotic-enhanced rehabilitation and virtual reality therapy to neurostimulation techniques and personalized medicine, the future of stroke recovery holds promises for tailored approaches that optimize recovery and improve quality of life. This chapter takes you into the emerging trends, breakthroughs, and potential challenges in stroke care, providing recent perspectives into the life-altering possibilities of technology in influencing the future of stroke recovery.

Evolution of Technology in Stroke Recovery

Over the years, technology has played an increasingly significant role in stroke recovery, leading to advancements and improvements in rehabilitation techniques and outcomes. Initially, stroke rehabilitation primarily relied on conventional therapies such as physical, occupational, and speech therapy. However, with the advancement of technology, new tools and interventions have emerged, revolutionizing the field of stroke recovery (Malik et al., 2022).

The Role of Technology in Stroke Recovery

Several kinds of technology are utilized during stroke recovery, including:

- **Robotic-assisted rehabilitation:** Robotic devices improve motor recuperation by supplying repetitive, task-driven workouts suited to personal requirements. These devices provide accurate control and feedback, enabling motion retraining and enhancing motor operation (Maceira-Elvira et al., 2019).

- **Virtual reality (VR) therapy:** VR technology places stroke survivors in computer-generated situations, encouraging interactive recovery workouts. VR therapy improves motor learning, motivation, and cognitive abilities, offering real-time feedback and tracking performance.

- **Neurostimulation techniques:** Transcranial magnetic stimulation (TMS) and transcranial direct current stimulation (TDCS) are noninvasive brain stimulations that modulate cortical excitability and encourage neural plasticity. These skills improve motor recuperation and cognitive function after a stroke (Maceira-Elvira et al., 2019).

- **Wearable devices:** Wearable sensors and accelerometers monitor movement patterns, gait, and balance in stroke survivors, providing real-time feedback and performance metrics. These devices promote self-management, adherence to therapy, and early detection of mobility impairments.

Emerging Stroke Technology

In addition to established technologies, several emerging forms of technology show promise in stroke rehabilitation and recovery:

- **Brain-computer interfaces (BCIs):** BCIs enable direct communication between the brain and external devices, allowing stroke survivors to control assistive technologies or prosthetic devices using their brain signals. BCIs can potentially restore motor function and enhance independence post-stroke (Malik et al., 2022).

- **Exoskeletons:** Robotic exoskeletons provide mechanical support and assistance to stroke survivors during gait training and mobility tasks. These wearable devices facilitate intensive rehabilitation, promote natural movement patterns, and enhance walking ability.

- **Artificial intelligence (AI):** AI-powered algorithms analyze large datasets, identify patterns, and personalize treatment plans based on individual characteristics and responses to therapy. AI holds promise for optimizing stroke rehabilitation outcomes through personalized, data-driven interventions (Malik et al., 2022).

- **Telemedicine and remote monitoring:** Telemedicine platforms enable remote delivery of rehabilitation services, allowing stroke survivors to access therapy sessions, consultations, and monitoring from the comfort of their homes. Telemedicine improves access to care, reduces barriers to rehabilitation, and enhances patient engagement.

Technology plays a pivotal role in stroke recovery by offering innovative tools and interventions that enhance rehabilitation outcomes, promote independence, and improve the quality of life for stroke survivors. As technology continues to evolve, the future of stroke rehabilitation holds exciting possibilities for personalized, adaptive, and accessible interventions that optimize recovery and well-being.

Virtual Reality (VR) Therapy

Virtual Reality (VR) therapy is increasingly utilized in stroke rehabilitation and recovery for its immersive and interactive nature, which enhances engagement, motivation, and outcomes (Maceira-Elvira et al., 2019). Here are five ways VR therapy is used and their benefits:

- **Motor rehabilitation:** VR environments provide simulated tasks and activities that challenge motor skills, balance, and coordination. Stroke survivors can engage in virtual exercises tailored to their specific needs, promoting motor learning, movement retraining, and functional recovery.

- **Cognitive rehabilitation:** VR platforms offer cognitive training exercises designed to address deficits in attention, memory, problem-solving, and spatial awareness post-stroke. Interactive tasks and puzzles in virtual environments stimulate cognitive functions and facilitate neuroplasticity, improving cognitive abilities (Maceira-Elvira et al., 2019).

- **Gait training:** VR-based gait training programs simulate walking scenarios in virtual environments, allowing stroke survivors to practice walking and balance exercises in a safe and controlled setting. These programs provide real-time feedback on gait parameters and promote confidence and independence in walking.

- **Activities of daily living (ADL) training:** VR simulations of everyday tasks, such as cooking, shopping, or navigating a home environment, help stroke survivors practice and improve functional abilities required for independent living. VR therapy enhances ADL performance, promotes problem-solving skills, and fosters confidence in performing daily tasks (Maceira-Elvira et al., 2019).

- **Psychological well-being:** VR environments offer opportunities for relaxation, stress reduction, and exposure therapy for managing anxiety, depression, and post-traumatic stress disorder (PTSD) following a stroke. Immersive experiences such as nature scenes, guided meditation, or virtual relaxation exercises promote emotional well-being and enhance coping mechanisms (Maceira-Elvira et al., 2019).

How to Use VR Therapy

Factors to keep in mind when using VR therapy in stroke rehabilitation include:

- **Safety:** Ensure that VR equipment is calibrated correctly and the environment is free from hazards to prevent falls or injuries during therapy sessions.

- **Comfort:** Consider individual preferences and comfort levels when selecting VR experiences and adjusting brightness, sound, and motion sensitivity to optimize comfort and immersion.

- **Accessibility:** Ensure that VR technology is accessible and user-friendly for stroke survivors with physical or cognitive impairments, providing appropriate adaptations or assistance as needed (Maceira-Elvira et al., 2019).

- **Therapist guidance:** VR therapy should be supervised and guided by trained therapists or healthcare professionals who can tailor interventions, monitor progress, and provide support throughout rehabilitation.

- **Integration with conventional therapy:** To maximize benefits and outcomes, incorporate VR therapy into a comprehensive rehabilitation program that includes conventional therapies, such as physical, occupational, and speech therapy (Maceira-Elvira et al., 2019).

Robot-Assisted Therapy

Robot-assisted therapy is used in stroke rehabilitation and recovery to provide precise, repetitive, customizable exercises that target motor impairments and promote functional recovery. Here are five ways robot-assisted therapy is used and its benefits:

- **Motor relearning:** Robotic devices deliver repetitive, task-specific movements to facilitate motor relearning and neural plasticity in stroke survivors. These devices offer consistent and controlled movements that optimize motor performance and enhance muscle strength, coordination, and range of motion.

- **Upper extremity rehabilitation:** Robot-assisted therapy targets upper extremity impairments, such as weakness, spasticity, and decreased dexterity, by providing interactive exercises and feedback. Stroke survivors engage in therapeutic activities, such as reaching, grasping, and manipulating objects, improving arm function and independence in activities of daily living.

- **Lower extremity rehabilitation:** Robotic exoskeletons and gait training devices assist stroke survivors in walking and lower extremity exercises to improve gait patterns, balance, and mobility. These devices offer mechanical support and guidance during gait training, promoting proper biomechanics and weight-bearing while reducing the risk of falls.

- **Feedback and monitoring:** Robotic systems provide real-time feedback on performance metrics, such as movement accuracy, speed, and range of motion, allowing therapists to track progress and adjust therapy parameters accordingly. This objective feedback enhances motivation, engagement, and adherence to therapy, leading to more effective rehabilitation outcomes.

- **Personalized treatment:** Robot-assisted therapy allows for customization of therapy protocols based on individual needs, abilities, and progress. Therapists can tailor exercises, intensity levels, and difficulty settings to optimize therapy outcomes and address specific impairments, ensuring a personalized and adaptive approach to rehabilitation.

Brain-Computer Interface (BCI)

BCI therapy is employed in stroke rehabilitation and recovery to facilitate neural plasticity, motor relearning, and functional recovery by enabling direct communication between the brain and external devices. Here are five ways BCI therapy is used and its benefits:

- **Motor rehabilitation:** BCI technology translates brain signals into control commands for external devices, such as robotic arms or computer interfaces, allowing stroke survivors to engage in motor rehabilitation exercises. Individuals can practice motor tasks and retrain neural pathways by mentally controlling movements, improving motor function and coordination.

- **Assistive device control:** BCI systems enable stroke survivors to control assistive devices, such as wheelchairs, prosthetic limbs, or orthoses, using brain signals. This promotes independence and mobility by allowing individuals to perform daily activities and navigate their environment more effectively.

- **Communication restoration:** For stroke survivors with communication impairments, BCI technology can facilitate communication by translating brain signals associated with language and speech into text or auditory output. This helps individuals express their thoughts, needs, and preferences, enhancing social interaction and quality of life.

- **Neurofeedback training:** BCI therapy provides real-time feedback on brain activity patterns, allowing stroke survivors to learn to modulate their brain signals through neurofeedback training. By practicing self-regulation of brain activity, individuals can improve attention, concentration, and cognitive function post-stroke.

- **Cognitive rehabilitation:** BCI systems offer cognitive training tasks and exercises to enhance cognitive functions such as attention, memory, and problem-solving. By engaging in brain-controlled cognitive tasks, stroke survivors can stimulate neural networks, promote neuroplasticity, and improve cognitive abilities.

Factors to keep in mind when using BCI therapy in stroke rehabilitation include:

- **Patient selection:** BCI therapy may not be suitable for all stroke survivors, as it requires intact cognitive function, adequate attention, and motivation to engage in brain-controlled tasks effectively. Assess individual capabilities and readiness for BCI therapy to ensure optimal outcomes.

- **Training and familiarization:** Stroke survivors require training and familiarization with BCI systems to control external devices or effectively perform brain-controlled tasks. Provide comprehensive training and ongoing support to facilitate skill acquisition and mastery.

- **Adaptability and customization:** BCI therapy should be adaptable and customizable to accommodate individual preferences, needs, and abilities. Adjust therapy parameters, feedback modalities, and task difficulty levels to optimize engagement and effectiveness for each participant.

- **Ethical considerations:** When implementing BCI therapy in stroke rehabilitation, consider ethical implications related to privacy, autonomy, and informed consent. Ensure that participants understand the risks, benefits, and limitations of BCI technology and have the autonomy to make informed decisions about their participation.

- **Integration with conventional therapy:** BCI therapy should complement and integrate with traditional rehabilitation approaches, such as physical, occupational, and speech therapy, to provide a holistic and comprehensive rehabilitation program. Collaborate with interdisciplinary teams to coordinate care and maximize therapy outcomes for stroke survivors.

Neuroplastic Research

Neuroplasticity refers to the brain's ability to reorganize itself by forming new neural connections throughout life in response to learning, experience, and environmental stimuli. This phenomenon allows the brain to adapt and compensate for injury, disease, or changes in function, playing a crucial role in recovery and rehabilitation after neurological damage such as a stroke.

Neuroplasticity research is just as important as therapy because it provides insights into the mechanisms underlying brain plasticity and informs the development of effective rehabilitation strategies. Understanding how the brain rewires after injury or disease helps therapists tailor interventions to promote optimal recovery outcomes by leveraging the brain's capacity for adaptation and repair (Malik et al., 2022).

Understanding Genetics

Genetic discoveries in neuroplasticity research have shed light on the genetic factors that influence brain plasticity and recovery from neurological conditions. Researchers have identified genes associated with synaptic plasticity, neurotransmitter function, and neuronal growth, which play critical roles in shaping the brain's response to injury and rehabilitation (Malik et al., 2022). By understanding genetics, researchers can:

- **Identify biomarkers:** Genetic markers associated with neuroplasticity and recovery outcomes can help predict individual responses to rehabilitation interventions, guiding personalized treatment approaches and optimizing therapy outcomes.

- **Develop targeted therapies:** Insights into genetic mechanisms underlying neuroplasticity inform the development of targeted pharmacological interventions and gene therapies to enhance brain repair and recovery after neurological damage.

- **Tailor rehabilitation programs:** Genetic profiling can inform the design of individualized rehabilitation programs that take into account genetic predispositions, allowing therapists to tailor interventions to maximize therapy effectiveness and promote optimal recovery outcomes.

- **Explore novel treatment targets:** Genetic discoveries open new avenues for exploring potential therapeutic targets and interventions to enhance neuroplasticity and improve functional outcomes in neurological conditions such as stroke, traumatic brain injury, and neurodegenerative diseases.

Appreciating the interplay between neuroplasticity and genetics is essential for advancing rehabilitation research and improving outcomes for individuals recovering from neurological conditions. By leveraging genetic insights and targeting neuroplasticity mechanisms, therapists can develop personalized, effective interventions that harness the brain's capacity for adaptation and promote optimal and functional recovery.

Advancements in Treatment

- Pharmaceutical advancements focus on more targeted therapies with fewer side effects and improved outcomes.

- Research into personalized medicine provides tailored drug regimens based on individual patient characteristics (Malik et al.,

2022).

- Emerging technologies such as telemedicine and digital health platforms are improving access to stroke prevention and rehabilitation services.

Noninvasive Brain Stimulation

Noninvasive brain stimulation is a technique that utilizes external means, such as electrical currents or magnetic fields, to modulate neural activity in the brain without surgery or invasive processes. This might include techniques such as transcranial magnetic stimulation (TMS) or transcranial direct current stimulation (TDCS). This approach helps patients by:

- **Modulating neural activity:** Noninvasive brain stimulation can enhance or inhibit neural activity by targeting specific regions of the brain, potentially improving cognitive functions, motor skills, and emotional regulation.

- **Promoting neuroplasticity:** Noninvasive brain stimulation has been known to encourage neuroplasticity, which is essential for recovery after a stroke or neurological injury.

- **Managing symptoms:** It can help lessen several neurological and psychiatric conditions, such as depression, chronic pain, and motor deficits.

It is thought to be a revolutionary type of therapy and rehabilitation because of the following:

- **Safety and accessibility:** Unlike invasive brain stimulation methods, noninvasive techniques are safer and more accessible to patients. They do not require surgery or implantation of devices, reducing the risk of complications.

- **Non-pharmacological approach:** It provides a non-pharmacological choice for enhancing brain performance and controlling symptoms, lowering the dependence on medications and their potential side effects.

- **Versatility and adaptability:** Noninvasive brain stimulation techniques can be easily adjusted and tailored to individual patient needs, making them adaptable for various neurological conditions and rehabilitation goals.

- **Research and development:** Ongoing research explores new applications and techniques in noninvasive brain stimulation, promising further advancements and refinements in therapy and rehabilitation approaches (Maceira-Elvira et al., 2019).

As Chapter 11 ends, we appreciate that we have taken a glimpse into the promising horizon of stroke recovery. It is true that the future beckons with creative therapies, better technologies, and a greater understanding of the brain's power to adapt. With researchers going beyond the limits of possibility, customized treatment schemes suitable for personal requirements are on the horizon. From virtual reality rehabilitation to neural implants, the environment of stroke recovery is constantly changing at an incredible speed. But in the middle of the excitement of the scientific revolution, only one truth remains constant: the undying resilience of the human mind. As we stand on the cusp of this new era, let us start on this path with hope, determination, and an absolute dedication to unwrapping the total capacity of stroke recovery.

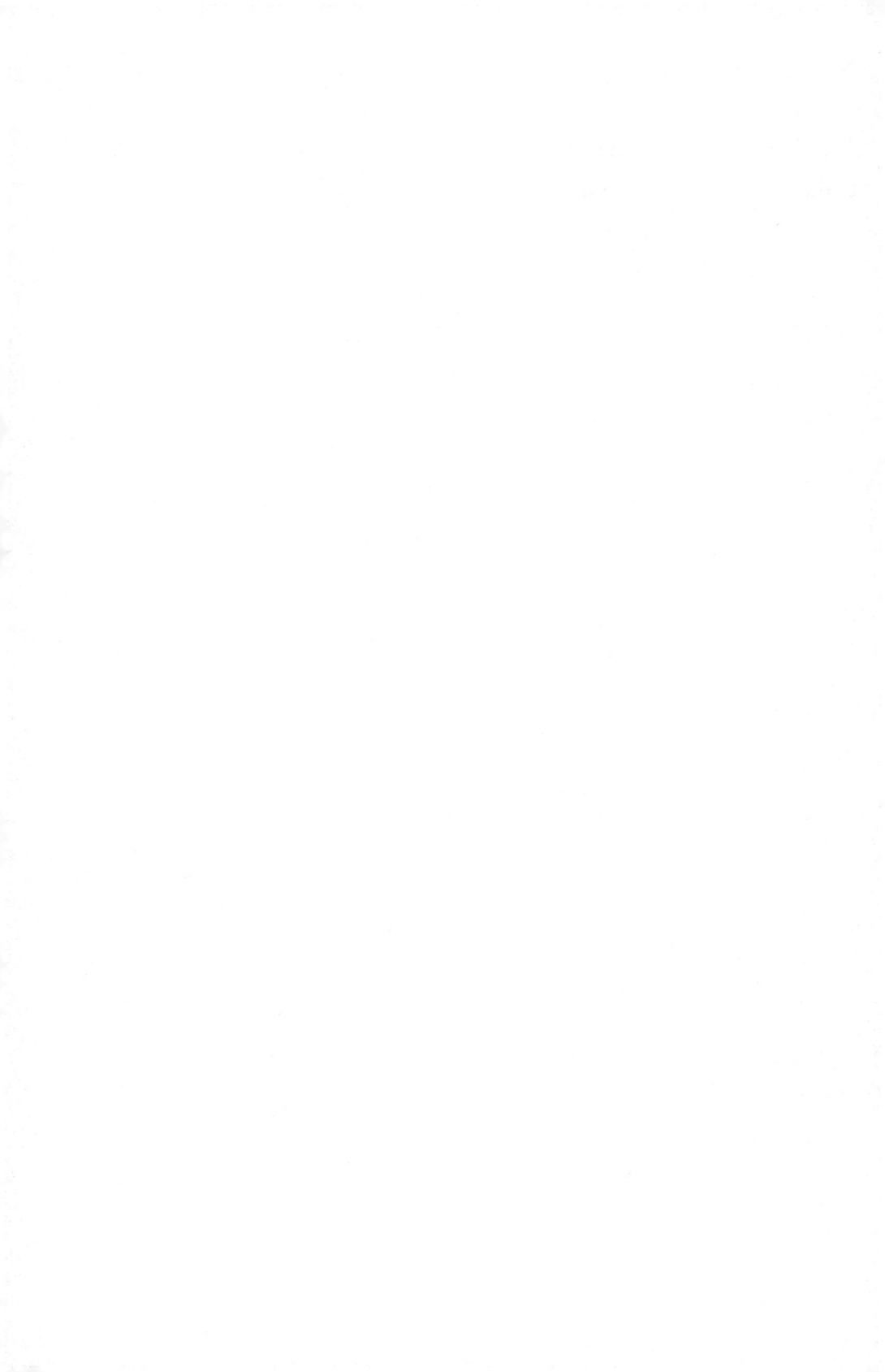

Conclusion

In concluding this comprehensive guide to stroke recovery through neuroplasticity and nutrition, reflecting on the resilience within each individual embarking on this journey is essential. Recovering from a stroke is a formidable challenge, but it is also an opportunity for profound personal growth and transformation.

Neuroplasticity underlies your ability to master new skills, heal after a brain injury, and embrace environmental changes. Intricate cellular and molecular systems, such as synaptic plasticity, neurogenesis, and alterations in neural connectivity control it. Gaining knowledge on neuroplasticity enlightens the brain's resilience and adaptive potential, clearing the path for creative therapies and interventions in rehabilitation and neuroscience.

Healing from a stroke is an intricate procedure that includes physical and mental components. Each development and achievement represents proof of the body's and mind's resilience. As the unidentified quotation implies, the brain is an essential component in this procedure.

There's an essential connection between brain wellness and dietary habits, particularly regarding learning and memory. The best possible performance of your mind is directly affected by the substances you eat.

Sustaining mental clarity while encouraging a healthy brain in general needs particular nutrients, including B vitamins, the antioxidants present in vegetables and fruit, and fatty acids called omega-3 present in fish.

As technology continues to evolve, so does the potential for innovative interventions and therapies to enhance recovery outcomes post-stroke. From robotic-assisted rehabilitation and virtual reality therapy to neurostimulation techniques and personalized medicine, the future of stroke recovery holds promises for tailored approaches that optimize recovery and improve quality of life.

As highlighted throughout this book, recovery is a deeply personal journey. No two individuals will experience a stroke or rehabilitation precisely the same way. Therefore, it's crucial to approach the process with patience, understanding, and self-compassion. Each step forward, no matter how small, is a victory worth celebrating.

The following are the key takeaways:

- **Holistic approach:** Embrace a holistic approach to stroke recovery, focusing on physical rehabilitation and mental and emotional well-being.

- **Neuroplasticity:** Harness the power of neuroplasticity to rewire the brain and facilitate recovery. Consistent and targeted rehabilitation exercises can help rebuild neural pathways and regain lost function.

- **Nutrition:** Nutrition is a foundational element of recovery. An unprocessed, whole-food diet rich in fruits, vegetables, lean proteins, and healthy fats can support brain health and well-being.

- **Patience and self-compassion:** Understand that recovery takes time and patience. Be kind to yourself throughout the process, celebrating progress and embracing setbacks as opportunities for growth.

- **Lifestyle modifications:** Make necessary lifestyle modifications to support recovery, including regular exercise, stress management techniques, developing and maintaining community and connection, and adequate rest.

In closing, remember that while the road to recovery may be challenging, it is also filled with moments of triumph and growth. You can reclaim your health and vitality by embracing the principles of neuroplasticity, nutrition, and self-compassion. Don't let your stroke define you—take the first step toward recovery; you will prevail.

My dear readers,

I poured my heart and soul into writing this book, investing countless hours and immense passion to create something truly special. It is my sincere hope that within these pages, you find insights, inspiration, and a sense of connection that resonates deeply with you.

Thank you for joining me on this journey. I genuinely hope that you gain something meaningful from this book.

Dr. Sterling

REFERENCES

Allatt, K. (2013, March 22). *Top 12 inspirational quotes that have INSPIRED me! Stroke Blog by Arockystrokerecovery.* https://arockystrokerecovery.wordpress.com/2013/03/22/top-12-inspirational-quotes-that-have-inspired-me/

American Stroke Association. (2019). *Emotional effects of stroke.* Www.stroke.org. https://www.stroke.org/en/about-stroke/effects-of-stroke/emotional-effects-of-stroke

Bailey, R. R. (2018). Lifestyle modification for secondary stroke prevention. *American Journal of Lifestyle Medicine, 12*(2), 140–147. https://doi.org/10.1177/1559827616633683

CDC. (2023, May 4). *Stroke treatment.* Centers for Disease Control and Prevention. https://www.cdc.gov/stroke/treatments.htm

Dongen, L., Hafsteinsdóttir, T. B., Parker, E., Bjartmarz, I., Hjaltadóttir, I., & Jónsdóttir, H. (2021). Stroke survivors' experiences with rebuilding life in the community and exercising at home: A qualitative study. *Nursing Open, 8*(5), 2567–2577. https://doi.org/10.1002/nop2.788

Foroughi, M., Akhavanzanjani, M., Maghsoudi, Z., Ghiasvand, R., Khorvash, F., & Askari, G. (2013). Stroke and Nutrition: A Review of Studies. *International Journal of Preventive Medicine, 4*(Suppl 2),

S165–S179. https://www.ncbi.nlm.nih.gov/pmc/articles/PMC3678213/

Hoffman, H. (2017, October 17). *17 ways to help stroke survivors recover faster*. Saebo. https://www.saebo.com/blog/17-ways-help-stroke-survivors-recover-faster/

Kirkevold, M., Kildal Bragstad, L., Bronken, B. A., Kvigne, K., Martinsen, R., Gabrielsen Hjelle, E., Kitzmüller, G., Mangset, M., Angel, S., Aadal, L., Eriksen, S., Wyller, T. B., & Sveen, U. (2018). Promoting psychosocial well-being following stroke: study protocol for a randomized, controlled trial. *BMC Psychology*, *6*(1). https://doi.org/10.1186/s40359-018-0223-6

Lee, M., Pyun, S.-B., Chung, J., Kim, J., Eun, S.-D., & Yoon, B. (2016). A Further Step to Develop Patient-Friendly Implementation Strategies for Virtual Reality–Based Rehabilitation in Patients With Acute Stroke. *Physical Therapy*, *96*(10), 1554–1564. https://doi.org/10.2522/ptj.20150271

Lin, T.-W., Tsai, S.-F., & Kuo, Y.-M. (2018). Physical Exercise Enhances Neuroplasticity and Delays Alzheimer's Disease. *Brain Plasticity*, *4*(1), 95–110. https://doi.org/10.3233/bpl-180073

Maceira-Elvira, P., Popa, T., Schmid, A.-C., & Hummel, F. C. (2019). Wearable Technology in Stroke Rehabilitation: Towards Improved Diagnosis and Treatment of Upper-limb Motor Impairment. *Journal of NeuroEngineering and Rehabilitation*, *16*(1). https://doi.org/10.1186/s12984-019-0612-y

Malik, A. N., Tariq, H., Afridi, A., & Rathore, F. A. (2022). Technological advancements in stroke rehabilitation. *JPMA. The Journal of the Pakistan Medical Association*, *72*(8), 1672–1674. https://doi.org/10.47391/JPMA.22-90

Maulden, S. A., Gassaway, J., Horn, S. D., Smout, R. J., & DeJong, G. (2005). Timing of Initiation of Rehabilitation After Stroke. *Archives of Physical Medicine and Rehabilitation, 86*(12), 34–40. https://doi.org/10.1016/j.apmr.2005.08.119

Mulhern, M. S. (2023). Cognitive rehabilitation interventions for post-stroke populations. *Delaware Journal of Public Health, 9*(3), 70–74. https://doi.org/10.32481/djph.2023.08.012

National Council on Aging. (2021, September 23). *The national council on aging*. Www.ncoa.org. https://www.ncoa.org/article/10-reasons-why-hydration-is-important

O'Dell, M. W., Lin, C.-C. D., & Harrison, V. (2009). Stroke Rehabilitation: Strategies to Enhance Motor Recovery. *Annual Review of Medicine, 60*(1), 55–68. https://doi.org/10.1146/annurev.med.60.042707.104248

Psychology, N. (2021, August 23). *Neuroplasticity, behavior, and dietary intake — rewiring the brain for better or worse*. Nutritional Psychology. https://www.nutritional-psychology.org/neuroplasticity-behavior-and-dietary-intake-rewiring-the-brain-for-better-or-worse/

Saunders, D. H., Mead, G. E., Fitzsimons, C., Kelly, P., van Wijck, F., Verschuren, O., Backx, K., & English, C. (2021). Interventions for reducing sedentary behaviour in people with stroke. *Cochrane Database of Systematic Reviews, 2021*(6). https://doi.org/10.1002/14651858.cd012996.pub2

WebMD. (2022, August 23). *Types of stroke: Ischemic, hemorrhagic, and TIA*. WebMD. https://www.webmd.com/stroke/types-stroke

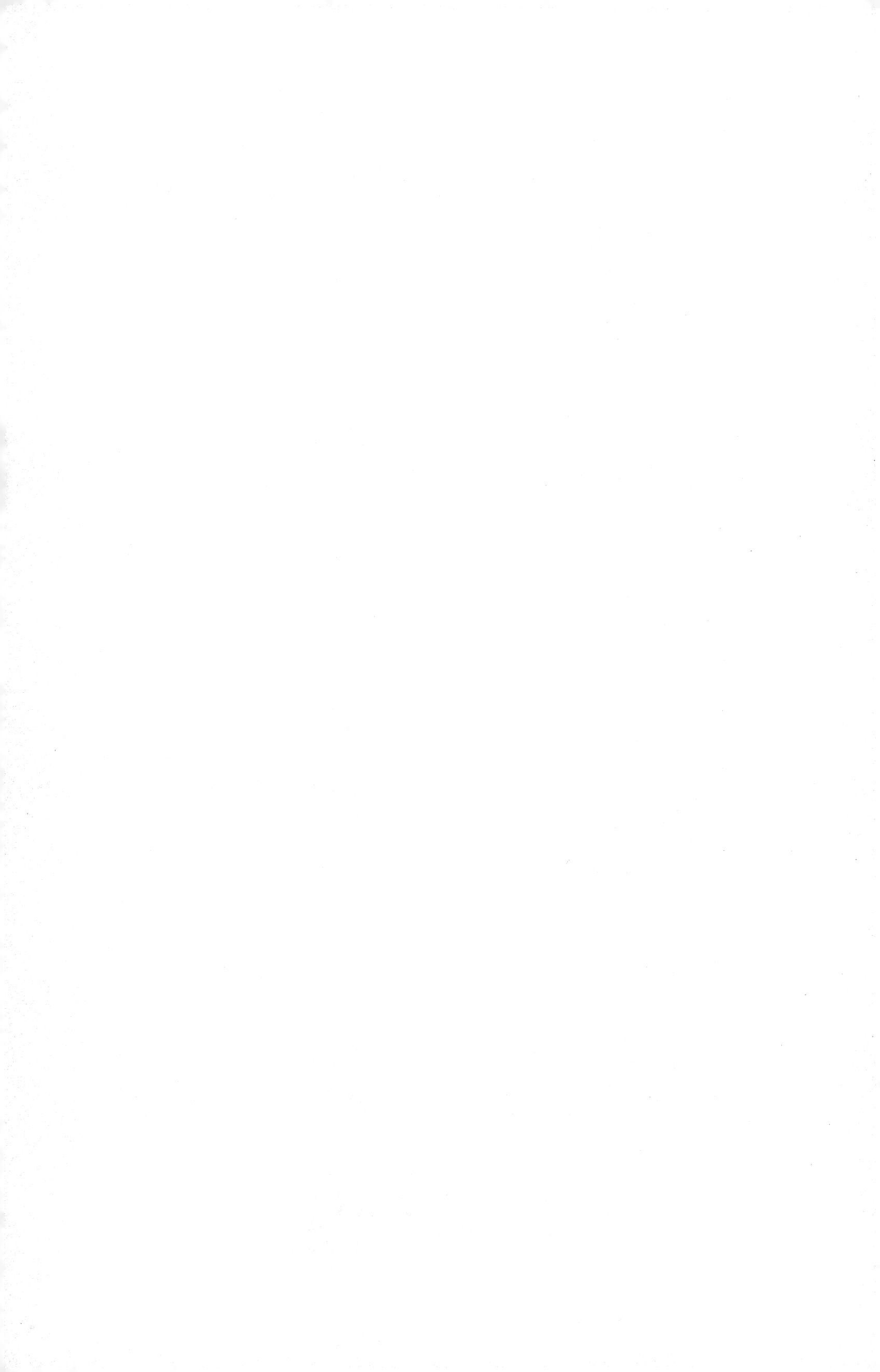

Made in United States
Orlando, FL
22 August 2025